Dr. Ann's Eat Right for Life™

W9-AVM-716

YOUR COMMON SENSE GUIDE TO EATING RIGHT AND LIVING WELL

By Ann G. Kulze, MD

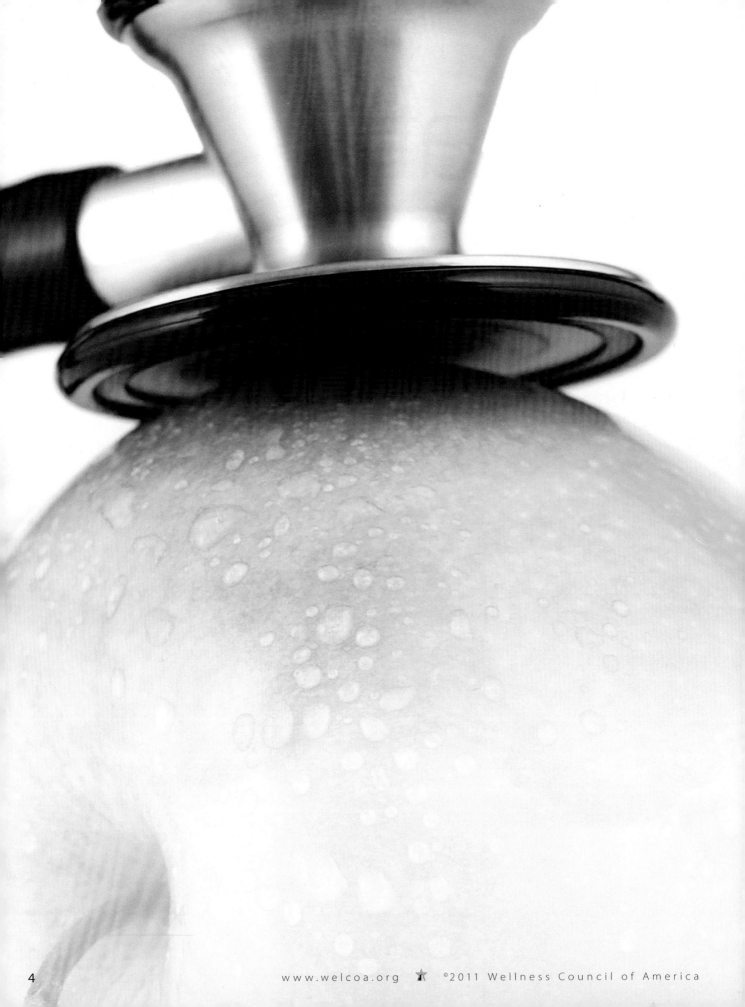

The Road Ahead

"…I have one simple mission—to teach you how to Eat Right For Life™…

…How can you get the most out of this book? Think of it as a devoted and caring friend. A best friend that is 100% committed to putting you on the pathway to radiant health…

…I want you to achieve nutritional excellence, but more important, I want you to experience the empowering feeling of being actively in control of your health…

…The way to good health is far easier than most imagine and holds a world of benefits that will stay with you for the rest of your life, so let us begin this amazing journey and take the first step together right now."

—*Ann G. Kulze, MD*

Editorial Staff

Author: Ann G. Kulze, MD

Executive Editor: David Hunnicutt, PhD

Managing Editor: Brittanie Leffelman, MS

Contributing Editor: Carie Maguire

Multimedia Designer: Adam Paige

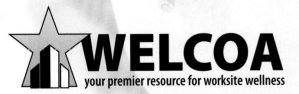

WELCOA
your premier resource for worksite wellness

17002 Marcy Street, Suite 140 | Omaha, NE 68118
PH: 402-827-3590 | FX: 402-827-3594 | welcoa.org

Dr. Ann
Ann Kulze, M.D.

Ann Kulze, MD
CEO
1 Pitt Street
Charleston, SC 29401
PH: 843.329.1238
www.DrAnnwellness.com

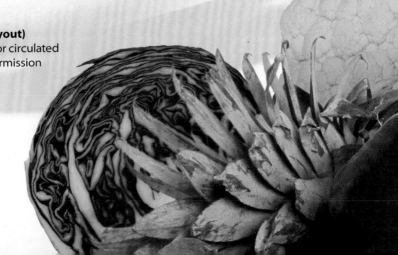

Table of Contents

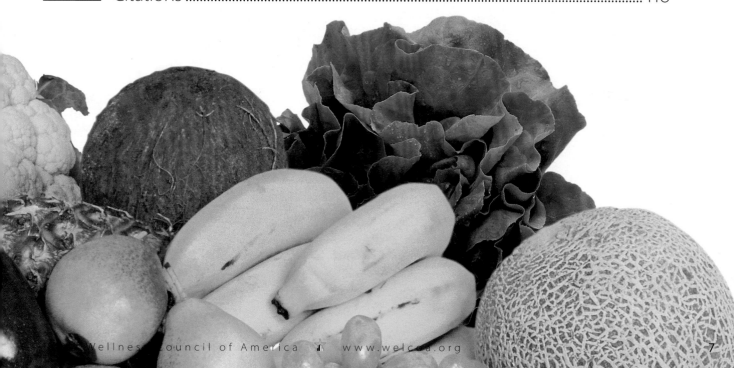

About **WELCOA**

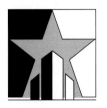

The Wellness Council of America (WELCOA) was established as a national not-for-profit organization in the mid 1980s through the efforts of a number of forward-thinking business and health leaders. Drawing on the vision originally set forth by William Kizer, Sr., Chairman Emeritus of Central States Indemnity, and WELCOA founding Directors that included Dr. Louis Sullivan, former Secretary of Health and Human Services, and Warren Buffet, Chairman of Berkshire Hathaway, WELCOA has helped influence the face of workplace wellness in the U.S.

Today, WELCOA has become one of the most respected resources for workplace wellness in America. With a membership in excess of 5,000 organizations, WELCOA is dedicated to improving the health and well-being of all working Americans. Located in America's heartland, WELCOA makes its national headquarters in one of America's healthiest business communities—Omaha, Nebraska.

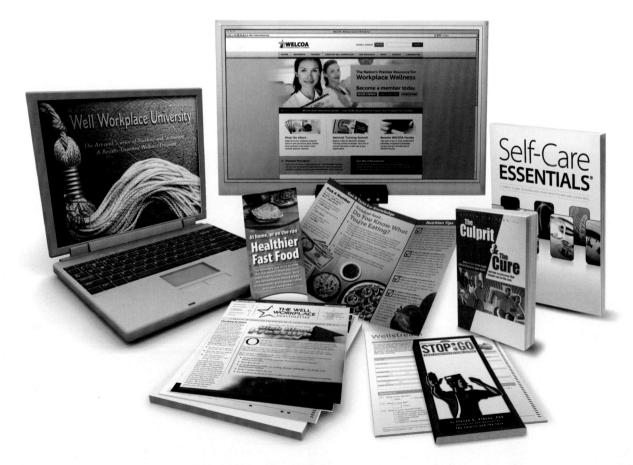

About **Ann G. Kulze, MD**

Ann G. Kulze, MD is a renowned authority on nutrition, healthy living, and disease prevention. She received her undergraduate degree in Food Science and Human Nutrition from Clemson University and her medical degree from the Medical University of South Carolina, where she graduated as the Valedictorian of her class. With formal training in both nutrition and medicine, in addition to her extensive "hands on" experience as a wife, mother of four, and trusted family physician, she has distinguished herself as a one-of-a-kind "real world" nutrition and wellness expert. She is the founder and CEO of the wellness education firm, Just Wellness LLC, and author of the books, *Dr. Ann's 10-Step Diet* and *Dr. Ann's Eat Right For Life™: Cookbook Companion.*

When she's not writing, researching, or motivating others through her speaking engagements, Dr. Ann lives her wellness message in her native Charleston, SC where she enjoys swimming, running, kayaking, cooking, gardening and spending time with her wonderful family. Learn more at **www.DrAnnWellness.com**.

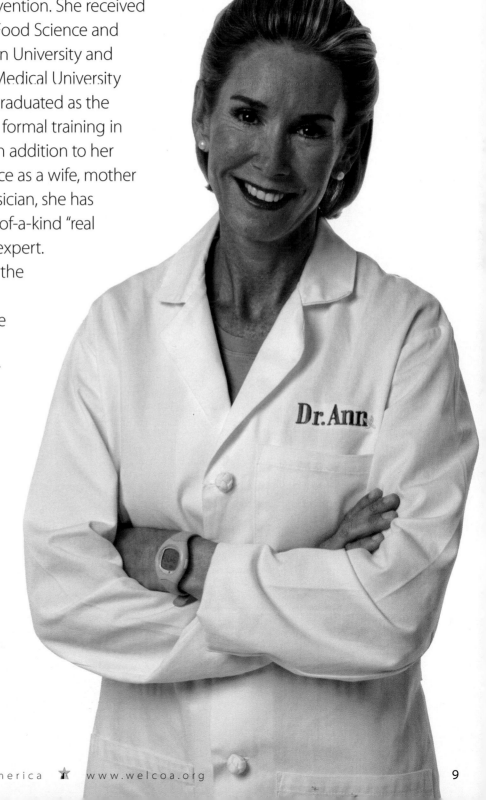

[FOREWORD]
From **Dr. Hunnicutt**

Each day, the typical person in this country will have to make more than 300 decisions about food. Although it sounds like a lot, it's just part of a normal day for most Americans. Now, if you are having a difficult time reconciling the fact that you'll have to make this many food-based decisions on a daily basis, you are not alone. In fact, I would venture to say that most people in this country have no idea just how many decisions have to be made—and therefore they discount the whole thing.

But let's take a closer look at what a typical day looks like for most people. Let's start with breakfast.

First, are you going to have cereal, toast, a breakfast bar, or just coffee and juice? If you selected cereal, what kind of cereal will you have? Oats, bran flakes, oatmeal? What type of milk? Skim, 1%, 2%, whole or soy? How big of a bowl will you have your cereal in? How much cereal will you eat? What size glass will you choose for your juice? Will you choose apple, grape, cranberry, or orange juice? Pulp or no pulp?

I think you get my point.

Without expert help and guidance, it's a foregone conclusion that the vast majority of people have virtually no hope in making the right decisions concerning food and nutrition. As a matter of fact, if you consume as few as 100 excess calories per day—the equivalent of one slice of cheese—you will gain 10 pounds per year. That's right— make one wrong decision out of the 300 and you could find yourself, over time, in a world of hurt. And make no mistake about it, the national statistics bear me out as more than two-thirds of Americans are currently overweight or obese.

But this need not be the case when it comes to you and your health. And that's why we've partnered with Dr. Ann Kulze to develop this tremendously helpful book: *Eat Right For Life*™.

I've known Dr. Ann for more than a decade. I've watched her work take shape, and her approach to helping America make better food choices is above reproach. To be sure, we couldn't have asked for a more qualified, more thoughtful, and more plugged-in perspective than Dr. Ann's.

We're thrilled to partner with her and I can assure you that you are going to fall in love with her passion and her approach to eating more healthfully. In fact, I would go so far as to say this: If you follow Dr. Ann's advice, you are going to make the rest of your life the best of your life.

For simplicity's sake, this book has been divided into five major sections—and each contains powerful tips and strategies to help you eat the foods that will keep you healthy. Section one provides expert guidance on how to choose the right fats. Section two examines which carbs will keep you moving forward and which ones will do you in. Section three zeroes in on the wonderful world of fruits and vegetables and how you can maximize the power of these great foods. Section four then demystifies which protein sources are best for you and your health goals. Last but not least, Dr. Ann tackles the topic of choosing the right beverages—you'll be astounded by what you read in this section.

When all is said and done, you will have at your fingertips the blueprint for eating healthy and living the life you dreamed of. With Dr. Ann as your guide, I can assure you your trip will be a memorable and pleasurable one—you won't find any empty promises or schlock science in this book.

In these challenging times, it's important that you know that both Dr. Ann and I believe in the power of good health, and we subscribe personally and wholeheartedly to the information contained in the chapters of this book. If you are looking to make some changes in your life, this book can help you. If you are looking to maintain your present good health status, by adhering to Dr. Ann's advice you can confidently make great health choices.

We're thrilled with the release of this book, we're thrilled with our partnership with Dr. Ann, and we're thrilled that you've chosen this as your guide to better health.

Warmest Regards,

David Hunnicutt, PhD
President
Wellness Council of America

About
Dr. David Hunnicutt

Since his arrival at WELCOA in 1995, David Hunnicutt, PhD has developed countless publications that have been widely adopted in businesses and organizations throughout North America. Known for his ability to make complex issues easier to understand, David has a proven track-record of publishing health and wellness material that helps employees lead healthier lifestyles. David travels extensively advocating better health practices and radically different thinking in organizations of all kinds.

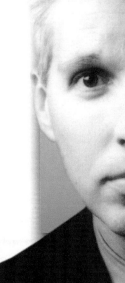

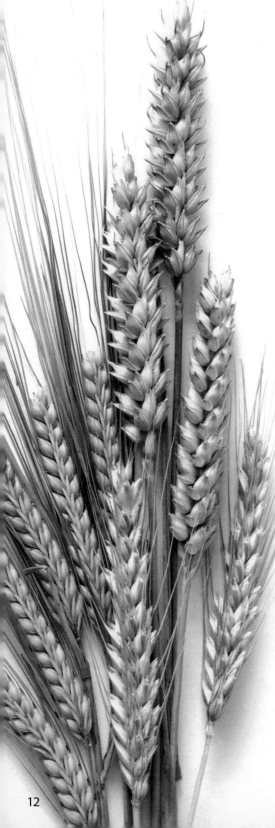

[INTRODUCTION]
Eat **Right** For Life™

If you want it to, this book can change your life. As a physician who has devoted her professional life to the science of nutrition, I want you to know the evidence is now irrefutable—you are what you eat. The foods you consume as part of a daily diet have a profound and lasting impact on virtually every aspect of your health and being. In fact, your diet is perhaps the single greatest determinant of your future health, not to mention your day-to-day vitality. Thanks to an avalanche of science published over the past two decades, we now know that the majority of illnesses and chronic diseases currently so prevalent in America are largely preventable, and in some cases fully reversible, simply by eating the right foods. Take a moment to consider this fact: just by eating certain foods, you can radically reduce your chances of becoming ill while transforming your overall health and well-being. This biologic reality is one of the most spectacular scientific advancements of modern times, and I am determined to help you take full advantage of it.

I have one simple mission—to teach you how to Eat Right For Life™. This book will guide you through the best ways to eat in order to maximize your body's extraordinary potential for radiantly good health. It is based on the most authoritative nutritional research available, but spelled out in a way that is both easy to understand and to follow. There have been hundreds of thousands of new studies regarding nutrition and health over the past few decades, yet when you distill them all down, what remains is a small handful of straightforward principles. All you have to do is learn a few basic guidelines, put them into day-to-day practice, and you will have mastered the art and science of optimal nutrition. I have simplified them for you into five directives: *1. Do Your Fats Right; 2. Do Your Carbs Right; 3. Eat Your Fruits And Veggies; 4. Select The Right Proteins;* and *5. Drink The Right Beverages.*

I have dedicated the last decade of my professional life to these five basic strategies—using every possible outlet and opportunity to teach and encourage others how to incorporate these dietary directives into their day-to-day living. My greatest pleasure comes from witnessing the dazzling effects of this nutritional empowerment. I have watched countless individuals completely transform their health and quality of life just by following this approachable and easy-to-understand guidance. From shedding lots of weight to reversing type 2 diabetes, reducing cholesterol, lowering blood pressure, and alleviating pain and fatigue, people are improving their health and vitality with ease and enthusiasm, and happily reaping its rewards.

And now you, too, hold the power! Right in your own grasp you have one of the most effective and scientifically validated means to feel great for good and stay well for life. By following the guidance in this book, you will be taking major strides towards chronic disease protection including having a healthier body weight, preventing heart attacks and strokes, avoiding diabetes, reducing the risk of Alzheimer's, warding off cancer—and that's just the beginning. Learning to Eat Right For Life™ will invigorate your body, lift your spirits, sharpen your focus, boost your energy, improve your self-esteem, and even revitalize your sex life, all the while still allowing you to enjoy the delicious foods your body needs and loves. What could sound more appealing?

What should you expect from this book? It might be easier to start by letting you know what you shouldn't expect. First, throw out the idea that a healthy diet means eating strange foods or depriving yourself of great tastes. This is far from truth. If anything, you will find that some of the tastiest foods on the planet are some of the healthiest ones you can eat, like roasted almonds, dark chocolate, berries, and avocados. Eating for health and eating to enjoy the pleasure food provides can definitely go hand in hand. This is the delicious reality I live every day of my life, and you can experience it too!

Second, don't expect to be hungry. In fact, expect the opposite. One of the greatest benefits of eating the right foods is appetite control. The very same foods that keep our arteries open, lower our blood pressure, give us long-lasting energy, and slow the aging process are also the most effective foods for keeping hunger at bay. This effect is of immense value because managing hunger is the Holy Grail for keeping a healthy body weight.

Third, don't think you will be set apart from your family by virtue of eating well at the table. As a working mother of four children, I know the challenges that come with family dinner. Have no fear; this is a pragmatic, totally adaptable plan, designed with your whole family's nutrition in mind. After all, what is good for you is also good for the people you love.

When can you expect to see results? This depends on how quickly you can incorporate the five steps into your daily life. Implement them at your own pace; but the sooner you can, the sooner you will experience their profound and far-reaching benefits. To list all of them would take up pages, but the most welcomed, immediate results include weight loss, a renewed sense of energy, sharper mental focus, improved mood, less aches and pains, and even a spike in your self-confidence. As you move further along, you will experience a host of metabolic improvements, including lower blood pressure, improved insulin sensitivity, better blood sugar metabolism, healthier cholesterol levels, and lower levels of inflammation in the body. These changes are what eventually translate to the sensational, broad-spectrum disease protection that eating the right foods can provide.

How can you get the most out of this book? Think of it as a devoted and caring friend. A best friend that is 100% committed to putting you on the pathway to radiant health. Just as you would a trusted mentor, rely on it regularly and often for inspiration and guidance. Read it, re-read it, and read it again. Highlight its text, dog-ear its pages, study it, and memorize its *"Plan of Action"* sections. Sleep with it, eat with it, take it to the grocery store, walk on the treadmill with it, and share it with others—whatever it takes to learn its lessons and embrace it fully and completely.

I want you to achieve nutritional excellence, but more important, I want you to experience the empowering feeling of being actively in control of your health. From what specific foods go into your mouth, to what groups of foods you should avoid putting in your grocery cart or on your plate, there is no feeling as rewarding as knowing that you are taking steps towards becoming a healthier person, for yourself as well as for the people who love you. The way to good health is far easier than most imagine and holds a world of benefits that will stay with you for the rest of your life, so let us begin this amazing journey and take the first step together right now.

—*Ann G. Kulze, MD*

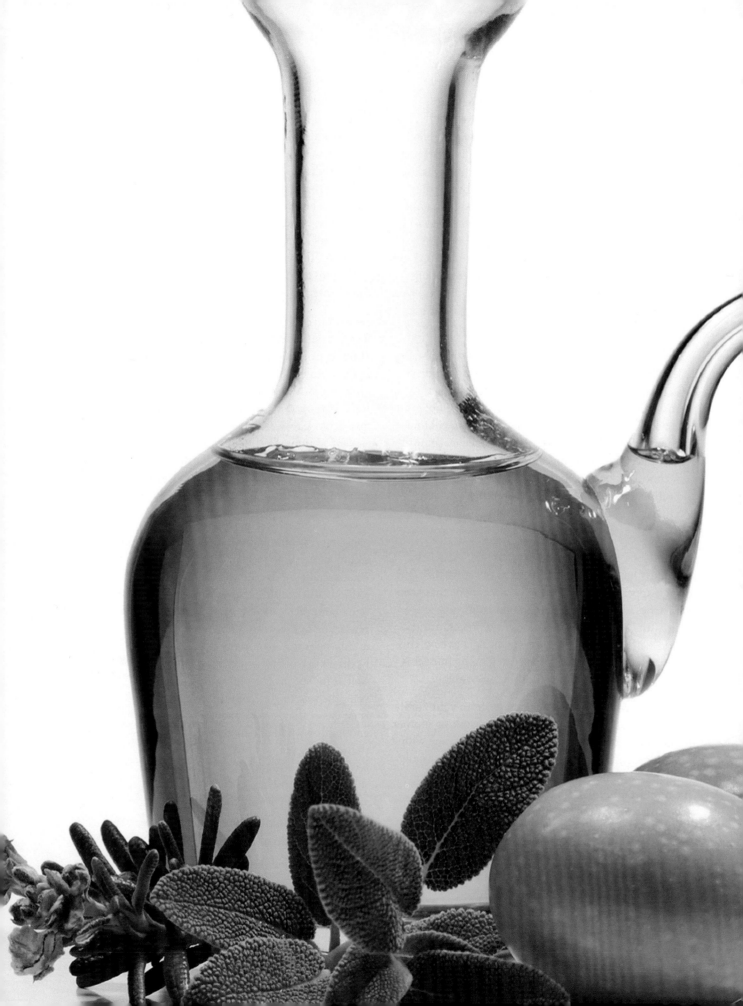

[CHAPTER 1]
Do your fats **right**

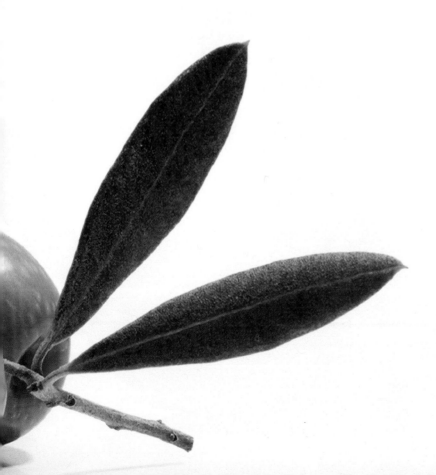

[CHAPTER 1]

Do your fats **right**

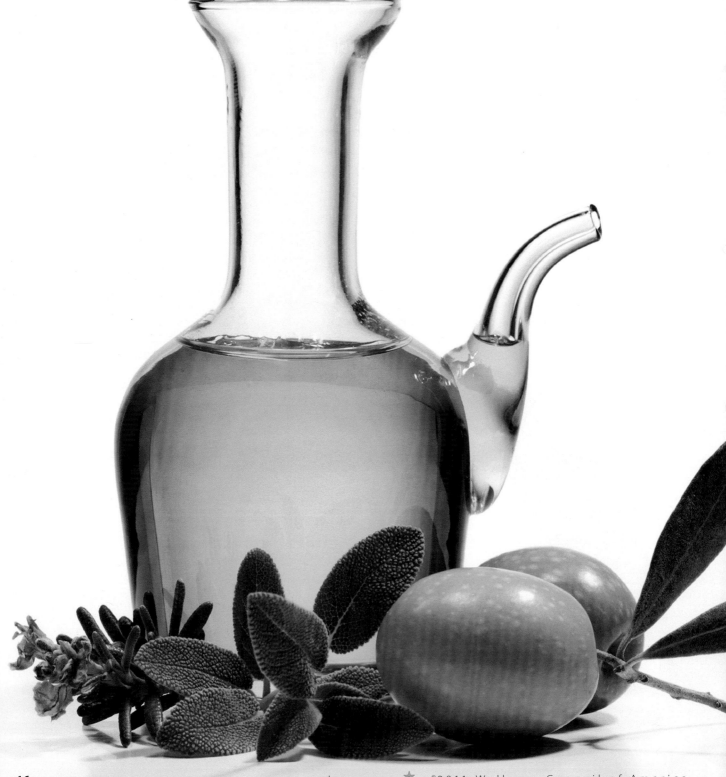

 www.welcoa.org ★ ©2011 Wellness Council of America

Of all the nutritional strategies that protect your health and improve your vitality, learning how to do your fats right is the single most powerful. This is a profoundly important statement, so I am going to repeat it to help emblazon it in your memory: Consuming the right fats, while avoiding the wrong fats, is the most important dietary strategy to guard your health and maximize your wellness. And now for some wonderful news—succeeding in this essential healthy eating directive is as simple as an oil change! Out with the bad and in with the good is all you really have to do.

The science is now very clear—when it comes to dietary fat and health, it's not so much the amount of fat that really matters, but rather, the type of fat. Some fats are positively, demonstrably great for you, while others are positively, demonstrably bad for you. Forget the "low-fat" dogma that was so heavily promoted and popularized in the 80s and 90s and wake up and taste the 21st century. Recommending low-fat diets is an archaic over-simplification of the scientific facts and throws the proverbial baby out with the bath water. So, have your fat and eat it too—just be sure it's the right fat!

This should be welcome news for those who consider eating one of life's greatest sources of pleasure. After all, it is largely fat that gives food its flavor and wonderful texture. I want you to fully experience the joys of eating while simultaneously improving your health. Learning how to do your fats right will give you this tasty and healthy opportunity. The name of the game is identifying and eliminating (or restricting) the bad fats while identifying and incorporating the good fats.

The Heart Of
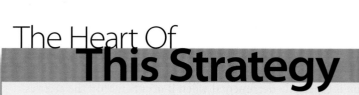
This Strategy

If you are curious why this particular nutritional strategy reigns supreme in the journey to good health, there is one simple and straightforward answer: It helps prevent and protect individuals from cardiovascular disease. Cardiovascular disease remains America's single biggest killer—taking more lives than all types of cancer combined. By choosing the right fats and avoiding the wrong ones, you can slash the risk of this notorious killer. And that's just the beginning. Doing your fats right also provides the following benefits:

- Improved neurologic and mental health
- Protection from some cancers
- Decreased risk of type 2 diabetes

- An improved blood fat (lipid) profile
- A more efficient metabolism
- Decreased inflammation in the body

I get especially excited about the last bullet, as we now recognize that excess inflammation plays a pivotal role in the development and progression of almost all chronic diseases—even the aging process itself.

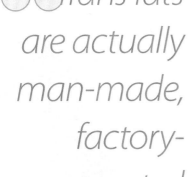

"Trans fats are actually man-made, factory-generated fats."

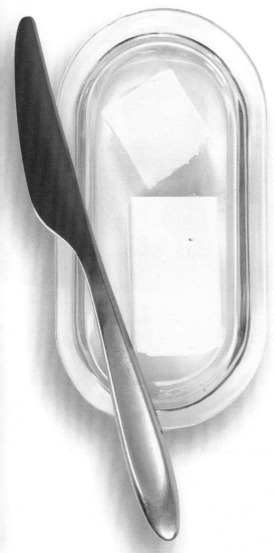

The Good, The Bad & The Hungry:
How To Leverage The Right Fats To Satisfy Your Cravings And Improve Your Health

There are essentially two categories of bad, unhealthy fats and two categories of good, healthy fats. As mentioned earlier, the key to doing your fats right is recognizing where the bad fats lurk, and eliminating them from your diet. And for the good fats—knowing what foods provide them, and bringing them into your diet. The remainder of this chapter will provide detailed information and strategies that will allow you to succeed with this. Let's go ahead and get the bad guys out of the way first.

THE TWO BAD FATS
Bad Fat #1: Trans Fats

Simply put, trans fats are poisons. They are truly toxic substances and represent the unhealthiest ingredient in our food supply. Think of them as the food equivalent of tobacco. There is no known safe limit for any amount of this sinister, noxious agent. I urge you to strive for a zero tolerance policy when it comes to trans fats.

Trans fats are actually man-made, factory-generated fats. They are produced from a modern food technology process known as hydrogenation. During this chemical process, liquid vegetable oils are infused with hydrogen to create a fat that is solid at room temperature—like the transformation of soybean oil into stick margarine. This process is beneficial to the food industry because it improves shelf-life and provides cheaper raw ingredients. However, it is a disaster for our health on a number of fronts.

The Toll Trans Fats Take On Our Bodies

Trans fats provide a quadruple insult to your arteries, (what I like to call "the rivers of life") clogging them more readily than any other ingredient ever identified in our food supply. Specifically, trans fats elevate LDL (bad) cholesterol, lower HDL (good) cholesterol, elevate triglycerides (another unhealthy blood fat) and directly incite arterial inflammation. And excess inflammation is especially detrimental when it occurs within the arteries. We have recently learned that inflammation is involved in virtually all developing stages of heart disease—from the initial build up of arterial plaque to the consummate heart attack.

The Harvard-based Nurses' Health Study offers great insight on just how horrible trans fats are for the "rivers of life." Subjects who substituted a mere two percent of their daily calories from trans fat with a healthier form of fat diminished their risk of cardiovascular disease by a whopping 53 percent. Moreover, a second report from this same study found that subjects with the highest trans fat content in their red blood cells (a marker for how much is consumed) were three times more likely to develop heart disease than those with the lowest levels.

Unfortunately, the heart and arteries are not the only victims when it comes to the detrimental effects of trans fats. A growing number of studies have linked these structurally bizarre fats to type 2 diabetes, metabolic syndrome and insulin resistance. Insulin resistance is the metabolic precursor to both metabolic syndrome and type 2 diabetes and a major contributor in the current obesity epidemic. Furthermore, a study conducted by researchers at Wake Forest University found that laboratory monkeys fed an experimental diet laden in trans fats (eight percent of their total calories) had higher blood sugar levels, more insulin resistance and gained significantly more weight, especially belly fat (the deadly type) than another group of monkeys fed the exact same diet and calories without the trans fats.

Finally, there is preliminary evidence that trans fats may even have a negative impact on our intelligence. A study conducted at the Medical University of South Carolina reported that rats fed a diet composed of 10 percent hydrogenated coconut oil (a common form of trans fat) made many more errors in navigating a series of mazes (a standard measure of cognitive function in rats) than the control group of rats fed the same diet without trans fats.

How To Eliminate Trans Fats

Thankfully, it is easier than ever to rid your diet of trans fats. This man-made fat is only found in three basic categories of foods:

- Processed foods made with partially hydrogenated oils
- Stick margarine
- Shortening

To avoid processed foods that contain trans fats, you need to do your due diligence with labels. Fortunately, a new regulation passed in January of 2006 mandated that all processed foods must list trans fats as part of the standard nutrition facts labeling. So, simply scan packaged food's "Nutrition Facts" label for trans fats. If any amount other than "0" is listed, don't even consider putting it in your grocery cart, much less your mouth! You can also double check for trans fats by reading the ingredient list for the words "partially hydrogenated oil." If you see these words in the ingredients, some level of trans fats is present—so beware.

Processed foods most likely to contain trans fats include the following:

- Baked goods, especially sweets like cakes and cookies
- Crackers
- Fried fast foods
- Chips
- Popcorn

(Continued on page 22)

The Last Nail In The Coffin For Low-Fat Diets

The largest clinical trial (the only kind of study that can really tell the truth) ever undertaken to evaluate low-fat diets put the proverbial nail in the coffin. This study followed over 49,000 women ages 50 to 75 for a period of eight years. The report was dubbed "revolutionary" and found that those consuming a low-fat diet experienced the same levels of heart attacks, strokes, breast and colon cancer as those who ate whatever they wanted. Interestingly, women in the study who chose to decrease their trans fat or saturated fat intake did experience a significant reduction in cardiovascular disease. Remember, it's the type of fat in your diet that really matters.

Simply put, trans fats are poisons. They are truly toxic substances and represent the unhealthiest ingredient in our food supply. Think of them as the food equivalent of tobacco. There is no known safe limit for any amount of this sinister, noxious agent.

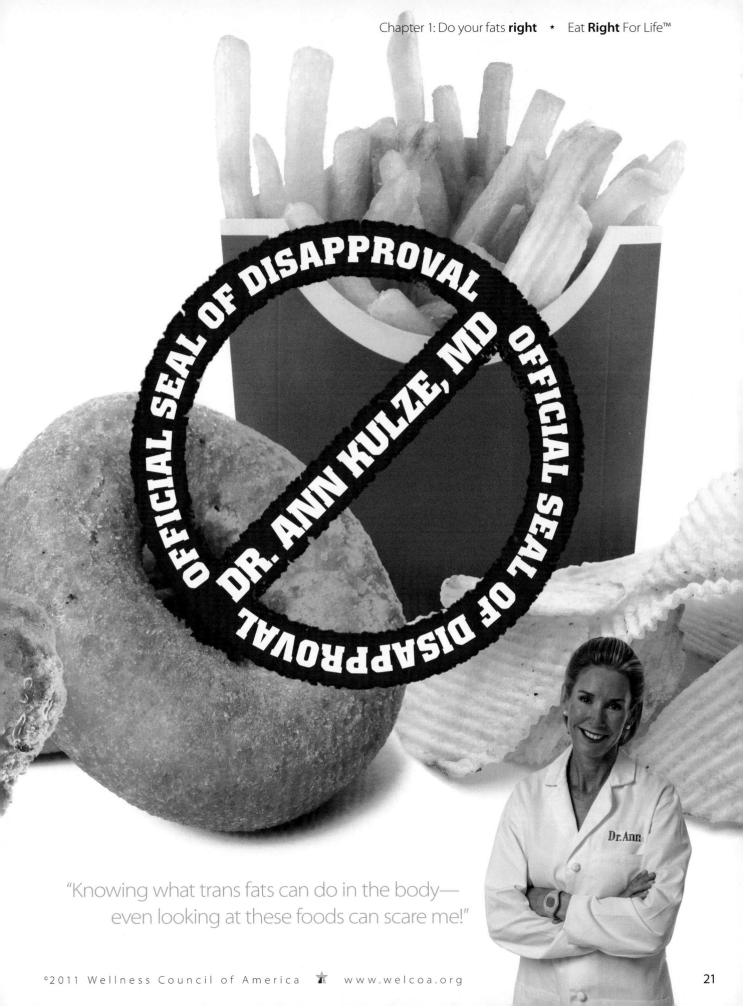

"Knowing what trans fats can do in the body—
even looking at these foods can scare me!"

Beware Of The "New" Trans Fat!

Many food producers are removing trans fats from their foods and replacing them with "interesterifried" fats. Emerging data has found that these fats may be even worse for us than trans fats. To identify foods that contain interesterifried fats, look for "fully hydrogenated oil" in the ingredients list.

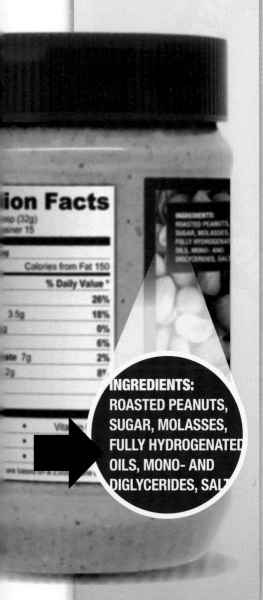

INGREDIENTS: ROASTED PEANUTS, SUGAR, MOLASSES, FULLY HYDROGENATED OILS, MONO- AND DIGLYCERIDES, SALT

It's especially important to note that some fast food chains and restaurants continue to fry in hydrogenated oils that contain trans fats. It's really best to forgo any restaurant fried foods unless you are sure it was prepared in a trans fat-free frying medium. The great news, however, is that since the trans fat labeling requirements were instituted, there has been a 75 percent reduction of trans fats in processed foods. The food industry has recognized that there is growing public awareness of the dangers of trans fats and that there are suitable, healthy replacements for this toxic substance.

Bad Fat #2: Saturated Fat

Saturated fat is the second type of bad, unhealthy fat. It's easy to remember what saturated fats are and where they're found if you think in terms of "four-legged fats." Meaning, the fats in four-legged animals, namely cows, pigs and sheep, are largely of this variety and can be found in red meat, whole dairy products (whole milk, full-fat cheese, cream etc.) and butter.

Like trans fats, these fats can clog your arteries. Indeed, saturated fats hinder the flow in "the rivers of life" by increasing your bad cholesterol levels. These four-legged fats slow the clearance of LDL (bad) cholesterol particles from the blood, and if that wasn't bad enough, saturated fats then directly stimulate the liver to make more of these particles. If you are among the 53 percent of adult Americans with an unhealthy cholesterol level, please make note that it is the saturated fat in your diet that is primarily raising your bad cholesterol levels. Relatively speaking, the cholesterol in your diet has a minimal impact.

Along with elevating artery-clogging bad cholesterol, saturated fats have been shown to impair the function of HDL (good) cholesterol particles. A recent study from the *Journal of the American College of Cardiology* added to previous evidence that even a single meal high in saturated fat can immediately impede normal blood flow. Investigators fed study subjects a meal comprised of 90 percent saturated fat and observed that it interfered with HDL (good) cholesterol's important job of shielding the inner lining of arteries from damaging inflammation. Ultimately, blood flow was diminished and clotting tendency increased. For someone with underlying heart disease, this scenario could be deadly.

Additional Effects Of Saturated Fat

The health risks of consuming saturated fat may not end within the arteries. In addition to the link between saturated fat, cholesterol and increased cardiovascular risk, eating high amounts of saturated fat has been linked to several chronic conditions, including type 2 diabetes, abdominal obesity, colon and pancreatic cancer, Alzheimer's disease and age-related vision loss.

There is also some new, intriguing science that demonstrates how saturated fats affect the brain and appetite. For example, when scientists infused palmitic acid—a specific type of saturated fat found in dairy and beef—

into lab animals, their brains sent signals to ignore appetite-suppressing hormones. Moreover, this effect was immediate and lasted for three days. Simple translation—cheese, fatty beef, butter and whole milk may literally change your brain chemistry, making you more likely to overeat for up to three days. Maybe you've noticed being exceptionally hungry on the Monday and Tuesday after a weekend bender of fatty food—this is a prime example of saturated fats at work.

How To Keep Saturated Fats At A Safe Level

Although saturated fats can have adverse effects, they are not "toxic" molecules like trans fats and are safe to consume in low amounts. It is easy to keep your saturated fat intake to acceptable levels if you adhere to the following three guidelines:

1. Limit red meat to two servings or less per week. Red meat includes beef, pork and lamb. Be especially vigilant in limiting fatty cuts of red meat like hamburger and processed varieties like bacon, hot dogs and sausage.

2. Restrict whole dairy products. This includes whole milk, full-fat cheeses, cream, cream cheese, ice cream, and sour cream. Instead, choose low-fat, reduced fat, skim and fat-free varieties.

3. Use butter sparingly. Opt for buttery-tasting spreads like Smart Balance or better yet, extra virgin olive oil.

66 ..be sure to check the label to ensure that it lists '0' grams of trans fat and is free of 'partially hydrogenated oil.' 99

A Quick & Easy Alternative For Margarine

In lieu of stick margarine, which is packed with trans fats, you can choose from a delicious array of "tubbed" spreads like Smart Balance. Whatever alternative you choose, be sure to check the label to ensure that it lists "0" grams of trans fat and is free of "partially hydrogenated oil."

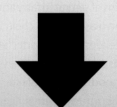

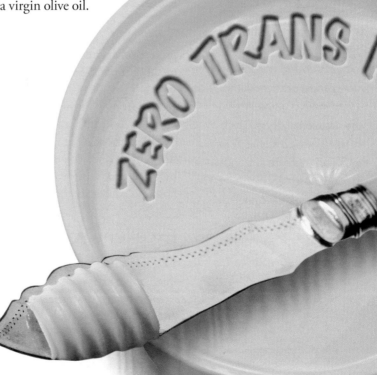

An Exception To The Rule:
Coconut Oil

Although coconut oil is a heavily saturated fat, it is an obvious exception to the saturated fat, four-legged animal rule. Coconut oil is different. Recent studies have indicated that coconut oil may actually have beneficial effects on blood fats. Coconut oil is uniquely high in shorter chains of saturated fatty acids, known as medium chain triglycerides. These shorter fatty acids appear to boost levels of good (HDL) cholesterol. Although definitive, long-term data on coconut oil and its impact on cardiovascular risk are not yet available, I'm comfortable telling you that coconut and coconut oil can be included in moderation as part of your quest to Eat Right For Life™. If you like it, enjoy shredded coconut in your granola or coconut milk in your Indian cuisine. When I very occasionally fry my chicken, I always use coconut oil as my frying medium. It stands up very well to very high heat and produces a wonderful crisp, finished product.

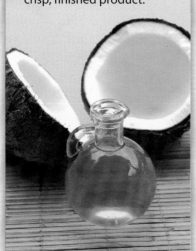

The Two Good Fats

Now that we have cleared your cupboards, shopping carts and ultimately your mouths of the wrong fats, we can replace them with the right ones. Indeed, including good fats in your diet can truly promote good health. The two good, healthy fats are the monounsaturated and omega-3 class of fats. The very best science available undeniably suggests that the majority of your daily fat calories come from these fats. Let's delve right into the tasty monounsaturated fats first.

Good Fat #1: Monounsaturated Fat

Monounsaturated fats are plant-based fats that remain liquid at room temperature. They can be found in olive oil, canola oil, avocados, nuts and seeds. When you include monounsaturated fats in your diet, you are literally guarding and improving your health. Just as you feel great about downing a plate of steamed veggies, you can feel just as empowered when you add monounsaturated fats to your diet.

The Big Benefits Of Monounsaturated Fats

So just how do these special fats improve and protect your health? In a nutshell (pun intended), they are the polar opposite of bad fats. Just as we learned how bad fats can clog your "rivers of life" and impair metabolism, monounsaturated fats can actually improve the health of your arteries and boost metabolism.

Monounsaturated fats help protect your heart. In fact, these fats can lower bad (LDL) cholesterol levels, lower triglyceride levels and in some cases even elevate HDL (good) cholesterol levels. Monounsaturated fats also offer some protection against insulin resistance, which can translate to a more efficient metabolism and protection from type 2 diabetes.

I know from working with thousands of patients that viewing certain high fat foods as healthy can be a challenge. After all, this is certainly a rapid departure from what many of us have heard for the past several years. To further convince you and send you on your monounsaturated way, here is a bit more about the healthy goodness monounsaturated fats can provide, and how you can easily incorporate them into your daily diet.

Excellent Sources Of Monounsaturated Fats

EXTRA VIRGIN OLIVE OIL

There is perhaps no other regional diet so powerfully and consistently linked to good health than the Mediterranean diet. Those enjoying this delicious and healthy fare usually live longer and have a lower occurrence of chronic diseases, including cardiovascular disease, Alzheimer's, type 2 diabetes, arthritis, autoimmune disease, some cancers and depression. Of course, olive oil plays a starring role in Mediterranean cuisine. Aside from housing the highest concentration of heart-healthy monounsaturated fatty acids, olive oil is also teeming with beneficial plant compounds called polyphenols. Polyphenols are potent antioxidant and anti-inflammatory compounds that exhibit truly eye-popping benefits in many lab tests. Preliminary findings show that polyphenols can help fight cancer, lower blood pressure, relieve pain and prevent blood clots. Although these laboratory findings have yet to be fully validated, it is now widely accepted that consuming foods with powerful antioxidant and anti-inflammatory properties is highly beneficial to your health. I consider extra virgin olive oil the healthiest oil you can eat because of its rich supply of heart-healthy monounsaturated fats and polyphenols.

The healthiest way to include olive oil in your diet is to use the "extra virgin" variety (EVOO). Extra virgin signifies that the oil has been obtained through gentle pressing of the olives as opposed to heat and chemical extraction. This process preserves its rich supply of polyphenols. Use EVOO in foods prepared or served cold, at room temperature or with low heat, like pan sautéing. Olive oil has a relatively low smoke point, (410° F) which means that if it is exposed to high heat (grilling, frying, broiling) its fatty acids become oxidized and transform into highly reactive, toxic molecules, called free radicals.

Quick Tips

Enjoy extra virgin olive oil in your salad dressings, dip your bread in it, drizzle it on your vegetables and pasta dishes after cooking or use a bit of it in your skillet before stir-steaming or gently sautéing your veggies over low heat.

CANOLA OIL

Canola oil, the other monounsaturated oil, is a relatively tasteless oil derived from rapeseeds. Canola oil provides a nice dose of omega-3 fats along with monounsaturated fats. This dynamic duo likely accounts for the truly remarkable results from the famed Lyon Heart Study. In 1988, French researchers took 605 adult survivors of a first heart attack and put half of them on the standard American Heart Association's "Heart Healthy Diet" and the other half on a special "Mediterranean Diet." The Mediterranean diet group included a specially formulated Canola oil-based spread as the primary fat. The study was initially intended to last for five years, but was halted after just two because of the profound benefits noted in the Mediterranean diet group. Those who followed this plan reduced their risk of death from any form of cardiovascular disease, including heart attack, stroke and heart failure by 76 percent.

Quick Tips

I recommend canola oil for dishes in which the high flavor of EVOO is not desired. For baking and high heat cooking, it's best to use "refined" also known as "high heat" canola oil, as standard canola oil has a lower smoke point and will oxidize readily when exposed to higher temps just as olive oil does.

The New Skinny On
Olive Oil

I consider extra virgin olive oil a superstar food, and a fascinating study in the October 2008 issue of *Cell Metabolism* provided yet another reason to make EVOO the oil of choice: appetite control. Olive oil is uniquely high in a specific type of monounsaturated fat called oleic acid. In this study, scientists infused oleic acid directly into the gastrointestinal tract of laboratory rats and found that it triggered the release of potent appetite-suppressive neurochemicals, which ultimately quiet the brain's hunger center. The laboratory rats that received the oleic acid ate less than the control rats that were not given the oleic acid. A similar report in *Gastroenterology* noted the same findings and also found that oleic acid delayed stomach emptying, giving rise to a prolonged sense of fullness. You can leverage olive oil's potential to quiet your inner cookie monster by incorporating the oil into your appetizers—try tossing a little extra virgin olive oil vinaigrette in your salad.

Discover more tips and tricks like these by watching a free video on my website:

www.DrAnnwellness.com

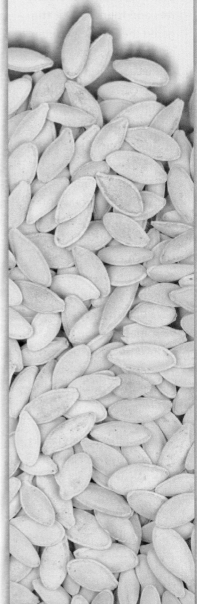

AVOCADOS

Avocados are exploding with life-preserving nutrients. I am always amazed by the number of people who consider avocados unhealthy or fattening. The reality is that this fruit is actually a true wonder food. In fact, avocados are included on the top 20 "most potent antioxidant foods" list. This unique fatty fruit provides a hefty dose of heart-healthy and metabolism-boosting monounsaturated fats that come along with a generous dose of fiber, vitamin E, B vitamins and special cholesterol-lowering plant agents called phytosterols. This unique package of nutritional attributes renders avocados extremely valuable for heart and brain health. Avocados are the quintessential brain food, so get smart and go guacamole!

Quick Tips

Avocados are a great addition to your salads. You can try mashing them and using them as a replacement for mayo on your sandwiches. Sliced or diced avocados with a little lemon and pepper are also delicious all by themselves.

NUTS

When it comes to life-saving performance, nuts score a perfect ten. They provide healthy vegetable protein, a rich supply of minerals, including magnesium, selenium and zinc, all forms of vitamin E, B vitamins, antioxidants and fiber, along with cholesterol-lowering phytosterols. They are also a superb source of the amino acid arginine, which provides the building block for the body's production of nitric oxide—the all important universal artery opener.

According to a number of powerful studies, including the Seventh Day Adventist Study and the Nurses' Health Study, consuming a small handful (about one ounce) of nuts five or more days a week can reduce the risk of death from cardiovascular disease by 30 to 50 percent. This is quite impressive considering that most prescription drugs only provide a 25 to 30 percent risk reduction (and they don't taste nearly as good!).

Concerns about weight gain from eating nuts regularly are completely unfounded. In fact, nuts are being studied as a possible "functional food" for weight loss. Cultures whose indigenous diets include nuts as a staple are leaner than their non-nut eating counterparts. And clinical studies back this up. With the exception of those who are allergic, I tell everyone—even those who need to lose weight—to include a small handful (about one ounce) of nuts in their daily diet.

In addition to pleasing your taste buds and protecting your heart, consuming nuts has been associated with a reduced risk of type 2 diabetes, vision preservation and longevity. *The Journal of the American Medical Association* reported that women who consumed an ounce of nuts at least five times a week were 27 percent less likely to develop diabetes versus those who rarely ate nuts. *The Archives of Ophthalmology* reported that consuming as little as an ounce of nuts a week reduced the risk of age-related macular degeneration, a leading cause of adult blindness, by about 40 percent.

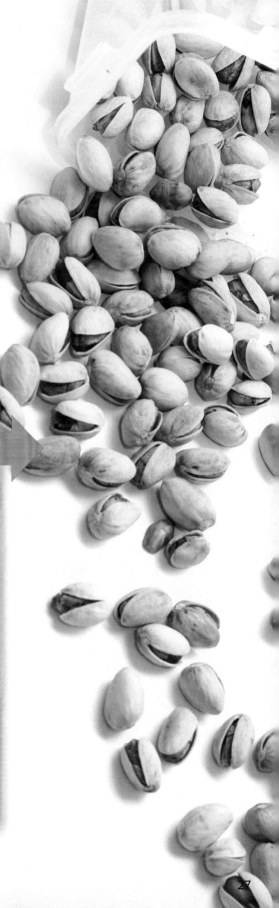

Quick Tips

You can choose from a variety of nutritious and tasty nuts, including cashews, walnuts, pecans, hazelnuts, almonds, Brazil nuts, macadamias, pistachios and chestnuts. Strive for variety as they each have unique nutritional features. For example, Brazil nuts are loaded with cancer-fighting selenium: walnuts are a great source of omega-3 fats: almonds are high in the potent antioxidant gamma tocophenol: cashews are loaded with copper and magnesium. Have them as your standard 4:00 PM snack. Throw them into your salads, top your oatmeal or morning cereal with a few or spread your whole grain bagel with some almond butter.

SEEDS

Like nuts, seeds provide a comprehensive and dense package of health-boosting nutrients and heart-healthy fats. Pumpkin seeds, sunflower seeds, sesame seeds and flax seeds can enhance the flavor of your meals or stand alone as a tasty snack. Furthermore, any oils derived from both nuts and seeds offer similar health benefits. Cooking with sesame seed oil, walnut oil and the like are not only healthy, but can also add interesting flavor to your dishes. Sesame seed oil and grape seed oil are great for high-heat cooking like stir-frying.

A Prescription For
Pistachios

Studies have repeatedly shown that nuts provide powerful cardiovascular protection. Although scientific evidence is firmly established for almonds and walnuts, studies on pistachios have been lacking. However, thanks to a clinical trial in the September 2008 issue of the *American Journal of Clinical Nutrition*, pistachios can now join the ranks as a heart-healthy food. In this study, scientists provided one, two or no dose (one dose = one small handful) of daily pistachios to three groups on equal calorie diets and measured the impact on their cholesterol levels. Those consuming the one and two doses of pistachios had a nine percent and 12 percent reduction in LDL (bad) cholesterol levels when compared to the no-pistachio control group after four weeks.

The study's authors concluded it was pistachios' unique "package" of nutrients and bioactive factors that were largely responsible for the results. Pistachios are an excellent source of healthy fats and are loaded with powerful antioxidants. Compared with other nuts, pistachios are the very best source of phytosterols (nature's cholesterol-lowering drug), potassium, vitamin B6, beta-carotene and lutein/zeaxanthin.

Don't Get Too Nutty:
Portion Control Is Key

Just as nuts and seeds are dense in nutrients, they are also dense in calories. Eat nuts or seeds daily, but limit your indulgence to one ounce—this is about 20 almonds or 12 pecan halves or roughly a nice handful. For those who are concerned about calorie intake, you can now buy pre-packaged, single one-ounce servings of nuts that give you "built in" portion control.

Good Fat #2: Omega-3 Fats

There are few nutritional topics that ignite my passion and enthusiasm more than the subject of omega-3 fats. Not only are these fats essential, but a flood of new data from the past two decades has revealed that they also have dazzling health benefits. Omega-3 fats are one of the most powerful weapons in our nutritional arsenal to defend against chronic diseases. However, as a result of modern food technology and agricultural practices, the availability of this fat in the standard American diet has dramatically diminished. Diets with insufficient amounts of omega-3 fats have been linked to several health conditions, including heart attacks, depression, arthritis, Alzheimer's, macular degeneration, autoimmune diseases, allergies and asthma. Conversely, higher intakes of omega-3 fats have been associated with protection from many of these same diseases.

The Big Benefits Of Omega-3 Fats

While monounsaturated fats like olive oil and canola oil are great for protecting your heart, omega-3 fats are hands-down heart health superstars. Hundreds of medical studies have demonstrated the powerful cardio-protective features of omega-3 fats. A powerful, comprehensive review of all published studies on the relationship between omega-3 fats and cardiovascular disease was published in the American Heart Association's Journal, *Circulation*. Based on this thorough evaluation, researchers determined that omega-3 fats provide seven separate cardiovascular benefits. These benefits include the following:

- Reduced progression of atherosclerotic plaque
- Reduced risk of arrhythmia and sudden death
- Lowered triglycerides levels
- Reduced blood clotting tendency
- Lowered blood pressure
- Enhanced arterial health
- Reduced arterial inflammation

Best of all: There are no dangerous side effects or prescription drug costs that accompany these benefits—all you have to do is simply eat tasty, omega-3 rich foods!

"In addition to pleasing your taste buds and protecting your heart, consuming nuts has been associated with a reduced risk of type 2 diabetes, vision preservation and longevity."

Omega-3 Fats: Then & Now

For our hunter/gatherer ancestors, omega-3 fats were plentiful throughout all areas of the food chain from tender green vegetation to fish to fowl and even large mammals like buffalo. In fact, paleo-anthropologists have quantified that our ancient predecessors consumed 5,000 to 6,000 milligrams of omega-3 fats a day. That is about 50 times more than the current average American intake!

The only good news in this tragic story is that omega-3 fats are left in so few foods that you can quickly and easily memorize the list:

- Oily fish: salmon, tuna, mackerel, sardines, herring and lake trout
- Walnuts
- Wheat germ
- Small leafy greens
- Whole soy foods
- Omega-3-fortified eggs
- Canola oil
- Flax seeds
- Oysters

Keep in mind that seafood and omega-3 eggs are the only omega-3 foods that can provide the biologically active forms, DHA and EPA. These two specific omega-3 fatty acids play direct roles in the regulation of our bodily processes. DHA and EPA are frequently referred to as the "long-chained omega-3 fats." Omega-3 eggs and seafood, especially oily fish, are the best food sources for this amazing fat.

Omega-3 & Heart Health

The scientific evidence supporting the cardiovascular benefits of omega-3 fats, DHA and EPA is so compelling that the FDA now allows food companies that provide products containing these fats to make claims on their package labels, promoting the heart-healthy benefits they can provide. As a result, more food manufacturers are spiking products like organic milk, salad dressings, margarine spreads and juices with DHA and EPA. Although every little bit helps, please know that the amounts of DHA and EPA in these "fortified" foods is typically much less than what you get in foods that provide them naturally like oily fish. For example, there are 100 mgs in some fortified milks, while there are 2,000 mgs in a two-ounce serving of salmon.

Omega-3 & Brain Power

The ancient Greek philosopher and physician Hippocrates was dead-on when he proclaimed, "What's good for the heart is likely good for the brain." If you take the human brain and remove all of its water, about 60 percent of what's left (known as the "dry weight" of the brain), is actually fat. However, the fat in our brains is nothing like the fat sitting on our hips and thighs, but rather a vital, structural, bioactive fat that plays a crucial role in all aspects of brain function (focus, memory, mood, etc). And it just so happens that the special fat that makes up the majority of the unique fatty architecture of our brains is none other than omega-3, specifically DHA. Think of DHA as your brain's most prized and highest quality building material. I like to refer to DHA as the "Fairy God Mother Fat" because it makes so many of our health dreams come true.

(Continued on page 32)

Heart Felt News For
Fish Oil

The Journal of American Cardiology recently gave omega-3 fats, DHA and EPA a glowing endorsement. After an exhaustive review of studies that included thousands of subjects, cardiovascular experts concluded that the data is "tremendous and compelling" that omega-3 fats in oily fish and fish oil supplements provide heart protection on several different fronts. Those who benefit most from omega-3's heart-healthy magic are patients with established cardiovascular (CV) disease who can enjoy up to a 30 percent reduction in CV-related death. The data also support heart benefits for healthy individuals too. The best dietary sources of DHA and EPA are salmon, herring, mackerel, sardines, lake trout and oysters. Fish oil supplements are also a simple and convenient option. However, it's always a good idea to check with your healthcare provider before taking supplements. To learn more about fish oil supplements and omega-3 fats, watch free video clips on my website:

www.DrAnnwellness.com

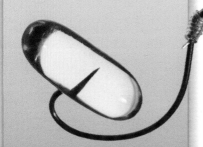

While monounsaturated fats like olive oil and canola oil are great for protecting your heart, omega-3 fats are hands-down heart health superstars. Hundreds of medical studies have demonstrated the powerful cardio-protective features of omega-3 fats.

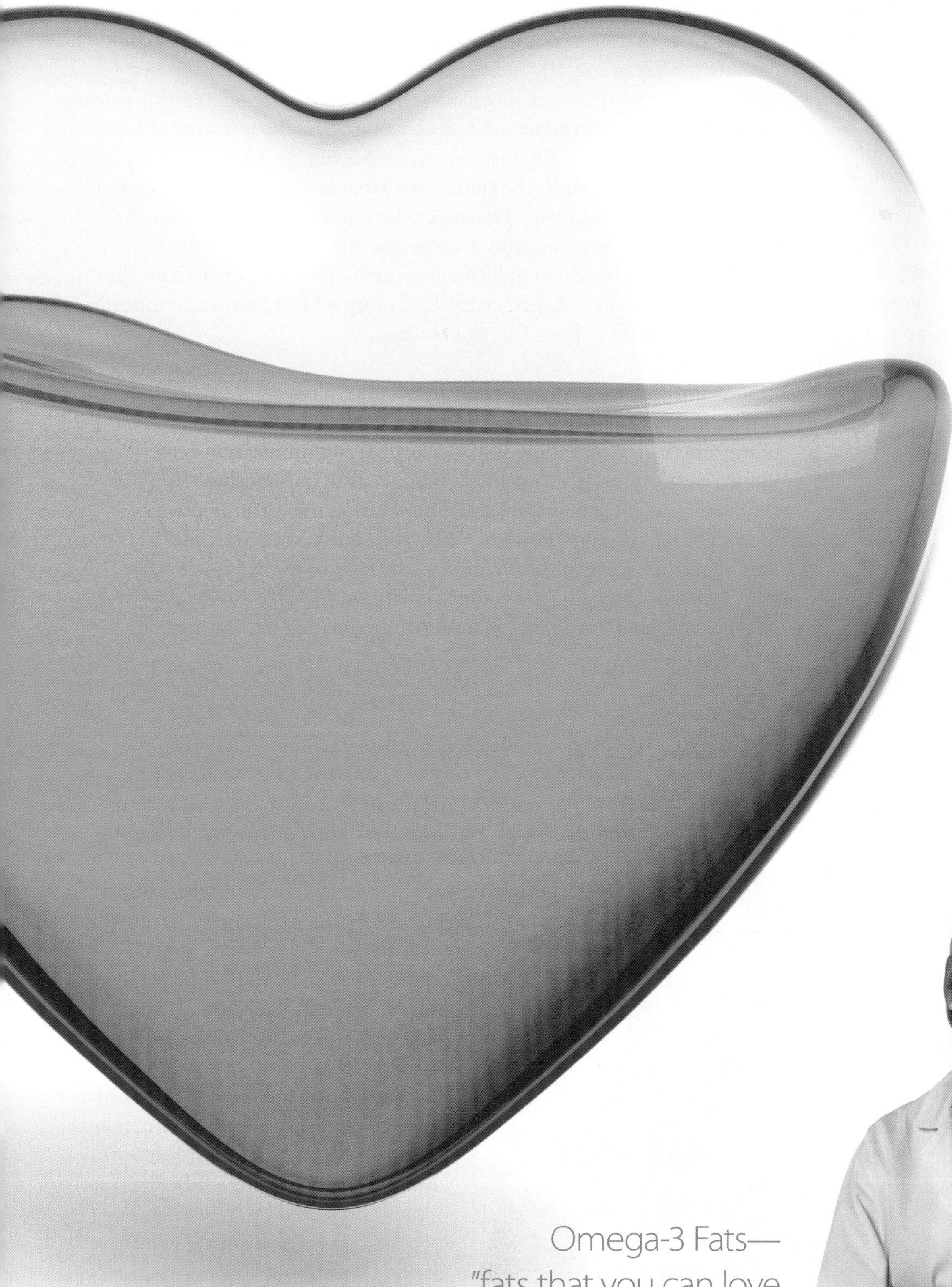

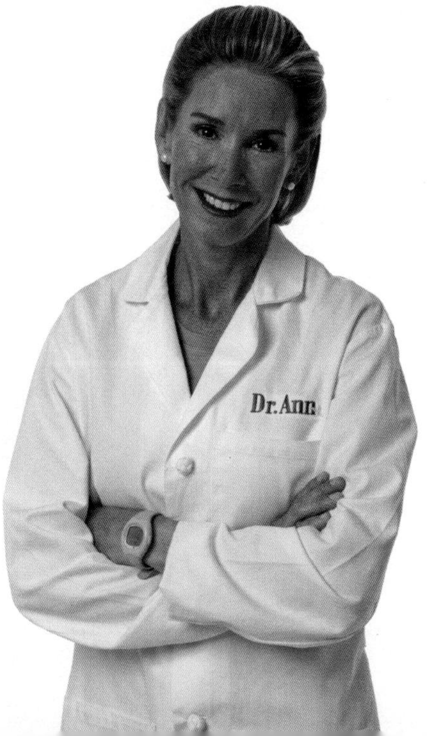

Omega-3 Fats—
"fats that you can love,
that love you back."

Pregnant Women Take Note:
Omega-3s Are Essential

The majority of the solid structure of the brain is formed in-utero, so perhaps there is no more critical time for getting optimal amounts of omega-3 fats than during fetal development. A report in the *American Journal of Clinical Nutrition* adds to other study findings that prenatal intakes of omega-3 fats via a mother's diet may boost her baby's brain power. In this particular study, 9-month-olds whose mothers had eaten DHA-fortified snack bars during pregnancy did much better on problem-solving tests compared to babies whose mothers had not eaten the DHA bars.

There are now algae-based DHA supplements available that have been specifically formulated for pregnant and nursing women. These supplements ultimately allow mothers to safely and conveniently consume optimal amounts of DHA during the critical period of gestation and infancy.

Considering the critical role that omega-3 fats play in brain health, and knowing that our intakes have so greatly diminished, it shouldn't really be a surprise that mental health disorders and degenerative neurologic diseases have substantially increased over the past 75 years. Repeated epidemiologic studies have shown a clear and consistent relationship between rates of depression and fish consumption. The residents of Japan are a brilliant example. Because fish and other omega-3 foods like soy beans are a dietary staple, the traditional Japanese diet contains about 10 to 15 times more omega-3 fats than the standard American diet. As such, Japan's rate of depression is about one-tenth the rate in the U.S. Further, a major review of published research looking at the relationship between depression and dietary levels of omega-3 fats found a significant antidepressant effect from this class of fats.

This "happy fat" appears especially important in both optimizing and preserving cognitive function. Indeed, the anatomic equivalent of learning is the formation of new neuronal communication centers known as synapses, which connect brain cells to one another. Think of the synapse as the lynchpin of learning. During the learning process, brain cells literally sprout or grow new connections called dendritites that deliver the learned information at the level of the synapse to the receiving cell. Dendrites are composed largely of DHA. Brains deprived of DHA are compromised in forming optimal nerve cell connections and thus learning.

A rapidly growing number of studies are shedding light on the fundamental role omega-3 fats (specifically DHA) provide for helping maintain intellectual capacities and protecting from the ravages of Alzheimer's and other forms of dementia. As part of the famed Framingham Heart Study, researchers collected data on the DHA blood levels in 899 adults. After following them for nine years, the people with the highest blood levels of DHA were 47 percent less likely to develop dementia versus those with lowest levels. In this particular study, those who had the highest DHA blood levels reported they ate fish two to three times a week. A second report found that healthy elderly men who ate the most fish had a slower decline in cognitive function than those who did not eat fish. Moreover, a provocative laboratory study conducted by researchers at LSU made history when they were able to identify just how DHA protects the brain from Alzheimer's

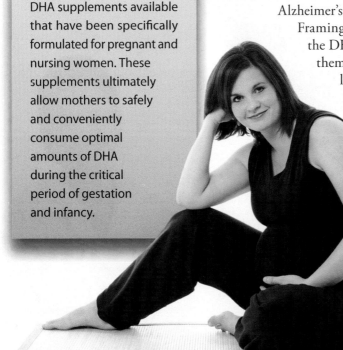

and dementia. They discovered that DHA actually reduces the brain's build up of damaging Alzheimer's plaques, by conversion to a substance called neuroprotectin D1. This protective agent, aptly referred to as the "golden brick," shields the brain from inflammation and oxidation, which can ultimately lead to Alzheimer's. Compared to normal brains, the LSU researchers found that some areas of Alzheimer's brains had 25 times less neuroprotectin D1.

Omega-3 & Our Overall Health

Let me give you one final reason to buy into omega-3 fats, and to buy in quickly: broad spectrum disease protection. It is now widely accepted that inflammation plays a pivotal role in the development of most chronic diseases. Heart disease and inflammation have long been tied, but we can now link excessive inflammation with high blood pressure, metabolic syndrome, type 2 diabetes, obesity, many cancers, Alzheimer's, Parkinson's, autoimmune conditions, allergies, asthma and even the aging process itself. Omega-3 fats are ferocious inflammation fighters. In fact, they are the building blocks for almost all of the body's innate anti-inflammatory substances. If you do not maintain optimal amounts of omega-3 fats, DHA and EPA, your body simply won't be able to effectively counter the damaging effects of excess inflammation. Therefore, eating omega-3-rich foods is one of the most effective strategies to keep your body's anti-inflammatory machinery in good working order.

Most nutrition experts agree that the average American diet is deficient in this critical essential nutrient. It's even been reported that DHA levels in the breast milk of U.S. women were lower than any other country except the Sudan. An additional study revealed that omega-3 fats couldn't even be detected in 20 percent of the study's participants. A few years back, I attended a conference at Columbia University that convened the world's experts on omega-3 fats and health. Joseph Hibbeln MD, a NIH-based renowned expert in omega-3 fats and brain health, was posed this question after his presentation: "What percentage of Americans do you think get enough omega-3 fats for optimal brain function?" His answer: "Perhaps two to three percent."

Bottom line: include omega-3 fats, especially DHA and EPA in your diet regularly. The richest food sources are oily fish like salmon, tuna, lake trout and sardines.

Omega-3 Fats Can Help You
Get Lean!

It sounds too good to be true, but emerging science suggests that omega-3 fats can help us lose weight. University of South Australia researchers divided 68 people who were obese or overweight into four groups. One group took daily fish oil (a supplement form of omega-3), the second sunflower oil (no omega-3), the third fish oil plus exercise and the fourth sunflower oil plus exercise. The group that exercised and took the fish oil lost an average of four-and-a-half pounds by the end of the three-month study. The sunflower oil group that exercised lost no weight as did the other groups that did not exercise. The lead researcher reported that "the omega-3 fats found in the fish oil likely increase fat-burning ability by improving flow of blood to muscles during exercise."

Quick Tips

Most nutrition experts, myself included, recommend 500 mgs to 1,000 mgs of omega-3 fats, DHA and EPA daily. (I prefer 1,000 mgs/day) If you eat three to four servings of oily fish a week, along with a few omega-3 eggs, you should easily meet this recommendation. If this is difficult or impossible for you to do, fish oil or algae-based DHA supplements are a convenient option. For those who are allergic to fish, algae-based DHA supplements like "Life's" brand are the best option.

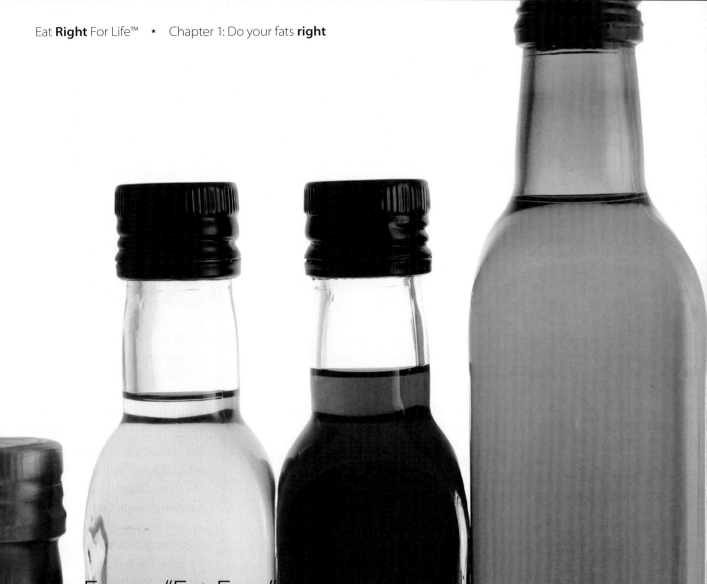

Forgo "Fat-Free"
Salad Dressings

Fat-free dressings clearly compromise the taste of your salad, but did you know that they can also compromise your health? In addition to providing flavor and texture, fats also act as a vehicle, transporting critically important, fat soluble nutrients, such as vitamins A, D, E and K. Fats also carry antioxidant phytochemicals like carotenoids from your digestive track into your bloodstream. With that in mind, it wasn't too surprising when the Harvard Nurse's Study found that women who put oil and vinegar on their daily salad slashed their risk of dying from a heart attack by 50 percent compared to those who used fat-free dressings. A second study had subjects consume a large salad with carotenoid-rich vegetables topped with fat-free dressing, reduced-fat dressing or full-fat dressing. The lead investigator reported that when people ate the salads with fat-free dressing there was virtually no absorption of the carotenoids. In contrast, both of the dressings containing fat led to increased blood carotenoid levels. Carotenoids are a class of disease-busting antioxidants that constitute one of the most powerful nutritional defenses plant foods can provide. They help prevent cancers, keep the cells that line our arteries functioning well, guard eyesight and protect our skin from the damaging effects of sunlight. Take full advantage of carotenoids by eating salads topped with dressing made with a healthy fat base (extra virgin olive oil is my top pick).

www.welcoa.org ★ ©2011 Wellness Council of America

I hope by now you are feeling informed, educated and motivated to do your fats right! I know this was a lot of information, so the following *Do Your Fats Right Plan Of Action* can help you remember and incorporate all of the necessary steps required for success.

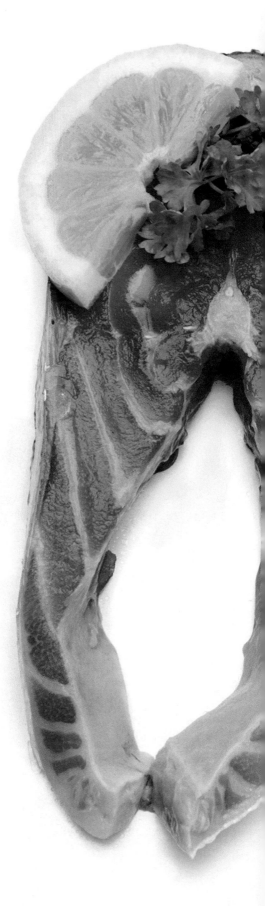

PLAN OF ACTION # Do your fats **right**.

1. GET THE TRANS FAT OUT COMPLETELY!

- Avoid stick margarine, shortening (Crisco) and foods containing partially hydrogenated oils (found in processed foods and fried fast foods).
- Only buy trans fat-free margarine spreads.
- Check nutrition labels: Look for "0" grams of trans fats on the nutrition facts label, and as a double check, scan the ingredients list—if you see "partially hydrogenated oil" listed, don't eat it!
- Do not eat fried fast foods—fries, burgers, chicken, fish, etc.

2. MINIMIZE SATURATED FAT

- Keep saturated fats to safe and healthy levels by abiding to the following:
  1. Limit red meat (beef, pork, lamb) to two servings or less per week. Consume the lean cuts (filet, tenderloin, etc.) when you do.
  2. Use butter sparingly. Enjoy trans fat-free margarine spreads (like Smart Balance) or extra virgin olive oil instead.
  3. Always choose reduced-fat, low-fat or non-fat varieties of dairy products over their full-fat counterparts.
- If you enjoy cheese and do not have a cholesterol problem, use the highly flavored cheeses (parmesan, feta, goat) or the less fatty cheeses (part-skim mozzarella and reduced fat cheeses) in moderation.
- Use Greek-style plain yogurt as a substitute for sour cream or cream cheese.
- Limit certain sweets. Ice cream is divine, but should be an occasional treat. If you love it, treat yourself once a week and know that some (ex: Ben & Jerry's) are much worse than others in regards to saturated fat content. I love Breyer's Light, Edy's Light, and Purely Decadent Coconut Milk ice creams.

3. CONSUME MONOUNSATURATED FATS AS YOUR MAIN FATS

- Use extra virgin olive oil or canola oil in food preparation—walnut oil, other nut oils and seed oils like sesame oil are also acceptable if called for in recipes. For cooking at high temps, use "high-heat" canola oil. For stir-frying, use grape seed or sesame seed oil.
- Consume nuts and seeds daily. Strive for a small handful (about an ounce) a day.
- Incorporate peanut butter, other nut-based butters and tahini (sesame paste); they are all excellent sources of monounsaturated fats.
- Enjoy avocados regularly—they are great for you!

4. GET THE OMEGA-3 FATS IN!

- Eat three or more servings of oily fish a week—salmon, tuna, sardines, herring, mackerel and lake trout.
- Enjoy walnuts, whole soy foods, ground flaxseed, wheat germ, canola oil, omega-3 eggs and dark leafy greens for additional omega-3 fats.
- Limit eggs to less than five a week if you are diabetic or have a cholesterol issue.

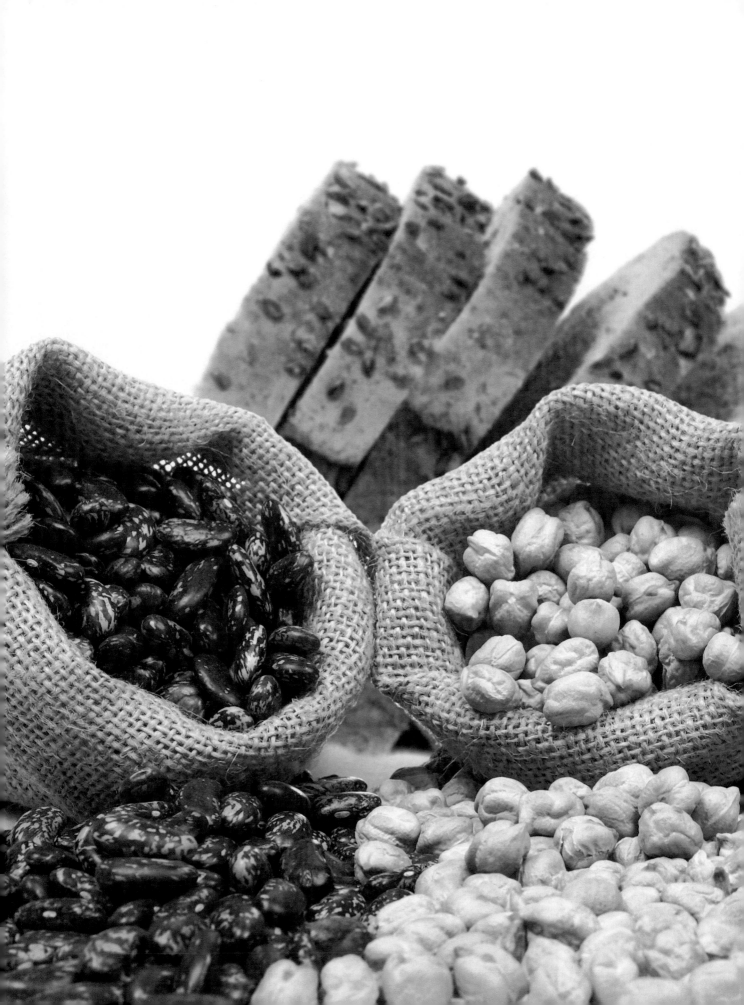

[CHAPTER 2]
Do your carbs **right**

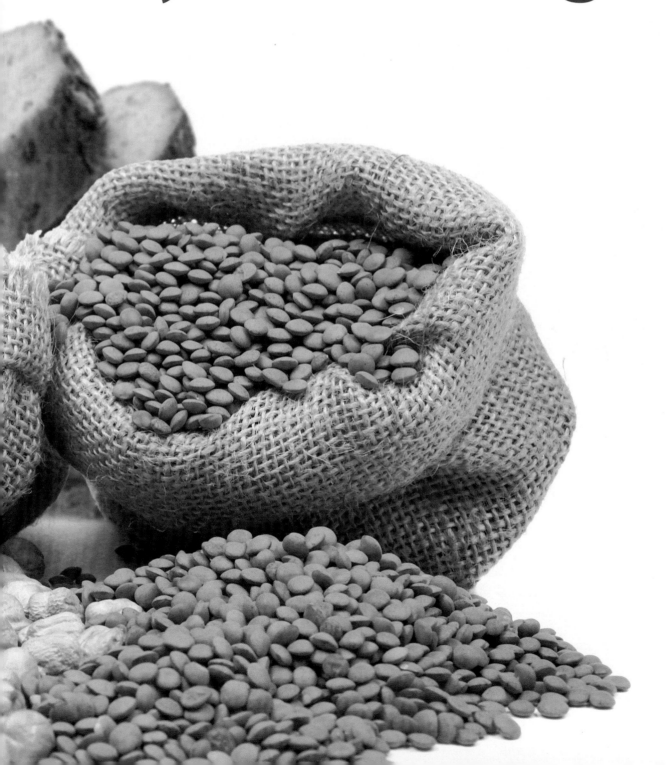

[CHAPTER 2]
Do your carbs **right**

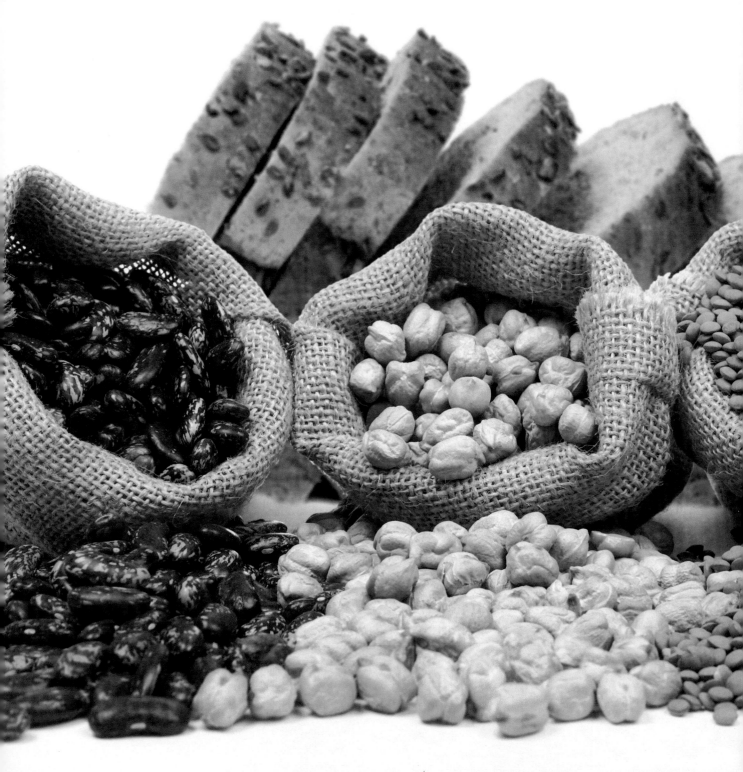

I t seems everyone these days is completely carb confused. Is bread good or bad for me? Can I eat sweet potatoes if I want to lose weight? Beans are starchy and fattening, right? With all of the carb-focused diet plans made famous over the past decade and the seemingly endless media coverage about this famous food group—how could you not be confused?

Thankfully, when it comes to carbs and your health and carbs and your weight, the facts are very straightforward. We are going to cover these facts in their entirety so by the end of this section you will be an expert—no more carb confusion!

First and foremost—forget low carb! Your simple task is to strive for the right carb diet. Have your carbs and eat them too, just be sure you choose the good ones. It makes absolutely no sense to eliminate foods that have been scientifically documented to help you manage your weight and stay healthy. Trust me, learning to do your carbs right is easy and delicious. It is also liberating and incredibly rewarding. In fact, this particular *Eat Right For Life*™ command closely follows doing your fats right as the most important eating strategy.

Just as with fats, there are good carbs and bad carbs. There is essentially one category of bad carbs and four categories of good carbs. In the end, the good carbs significantly outnumber the bad, so don't worry about eschewing the bad ones; there are many tasty, healthy and convenient carbs to enjoy.

Just as we did with the fats, let's go ahead and get the bad carbs out of the way first.

Clearing Up Some Carb
Confusion

For many decades, scientists have known that all carbs ultimately end up in your bloodstream as the same thing—namely glucose or blood sugar. In other words, the final common breakdown or digestive product of all carb foods is glucose. Whether you eat an apple, an orange, white bread, wheat bread, broccoli, carrots, French fries or sugar straight out of the bowl—it will all eventually end up in your bloodstream as the simple sugar glucose.

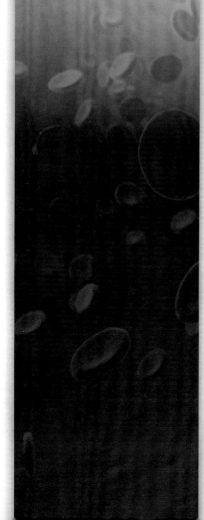

The Bad Carbs

It's very simple to identify the bad carbs because they are all white. This notorious group of carbs includes white flour products, white rice, white potatoes and sugar. Scientifically, they are known as the highly refined, high glycemic carbs. However, I refer to them as the "Great White Hazards."

This particular group of carbs has been repeatedly linked to a long list of adverse outcomes, including weight gain, cardiovascular disease, type 2 diabetes and even some cancers. I am sure you are wondering, "Dr. Ann, how can it be that the great staple of the American diet is so bad for me?" Don't worry, I am going to tell you the story in its entirety and in a way I know you will really "get."

Having practiced family medicine for 15 years, perhaps the single greatest piece of wisdom I garnered in working with my wonderful patients was that the "why" behind my directives and recommendations was what ultimately motivated them to follow through. I learned that it is not enough to tell people what to do and what not to do. Indeed, a clear, thorough and understandable explanation of the "why" is absolutely required. I want you to understand exactly how the Great White Hazards can lead to weight gain and just how they promote certain chronic diseases.

A Discovery That Changed How We Look At Carbs

In the early 1980s, a group of scientists made a truly revolutionary observation—it sent a seismic shock wave through the nutrition science community and we are still reeling from it. Specifically, scientists learned that, depending upon the chemical and physical structure of a given carb, there can be a vast difference in the amount of time the human body takes to digest it. The real shocker was when they discovered that many of the "complex" carbs like white bread, white rice and white potatoes were the very ones that were so rapidly and so easily digested. All these years, we considered these foods benign, healthy, and wholesome, and they are actually quite the opposite.

As mentioned earlier, we refer to quickly digested carbs as high glycemic carbs. All of the Great White Hazards have a high glycemic index. High glycemic carbs cause a sudden and dramatic elevation in blood sugar, which can lead to several problems, which again are weight gain, cardiovascular disease, type 2 diabetes and even cancer.

As nutrition experts, we're not just randomly picking on this group of foods. Indeed, we discriminate against this group strictly due to its glycemic response, which has been proven to cause metabolic stress. Some of the Great White Hazards (like baked russet potatoes) have such a high glycemic response that they can enter your bloodstream faster than if you ate sugar straight from the bowl!

See White: Think Fat

Now that you have scientific background on the glycemic response of the Great White Hazards, I can explain how they can make you fat. I'll use the popular fat-free white bagel (basically 100 percent white flour) to illustrate:

- You eat the white bagel and your digestive system quickly breaks it down.
- Glucose rapidly enters your bloodstream, sending your blood glucose level soaring.
- Your pancreas releases a corresponding surge of insulin— this is the point at which weight problems arise.

No matter what level of glucose enters your bloodstream, shortly thereafter a matching amount of insulin is released. Insulin is a fat-loving, fat-storing anabolic hormone. When insulin is released into your bloodstream, especially at high levels, it directs your body to store energy and deposit fat. To make matters even worse, high levels of insulin also block the hormone glucagon, which is a fat-burning and fuel-burning hormone. So, high blood insulin levels actually throw the body into fat-storage mode. Further, you cannot oxidize (burn) body fat when excessive insulin is in your system. When you eat the Great White Hazards, you will ultimately have a lot of insulin in your system.

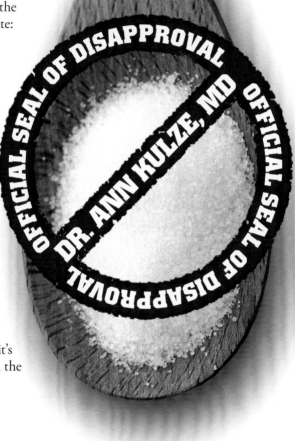

There is a second way the Great White Hazards lead to weight gain and it's even more powerful than the first. Let's go back to where we left off with the fat-free white bagel:

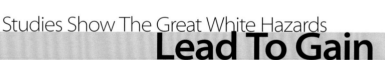

Eat white bagel ➡ blood glucose spikes ➡ blood insulin spikes

Studies Show The Great White Hazards
Lead To Gain

The Great White Hazards' propensity to boost appetite has been elegantly demonstrated in numerous controlled studies. Perhaps the most compelling was a study by Harvard's preeminent childhood obesity expert, Dr. David Ludwig. For this particular study, Dr. Ludwig and his team fed a group of obese 12-year-old boys identical breakfast and lunch meals on three separate occasions. The two identical test meals had a high, medium or low glycemic index. The high glycemic index test meals consisted of sweetened instant oatmeal, the medium index meals were steel-cut oats and the low index meals were veggie omelets with fruit. Although all of the different test meals had an identical number of calories, the study subjects ate 51 percent more food after the medium index meals and a whopping 81 percent more after the high index meals. The investigators clearly documented that the rapid rise in blood glucose levels after the high-glycemic meals induced a cascade of hormonal and metabolic changes that promoted appetite and subsequent food intake in this group of overweight study subjects.

A second study conducted to investigate the role carbohydrates play in obesity found that among 572 healthy study subjects, those who were heaviest reported eating the most refined carbohydrates. It's more than just coincidence that as waist lines have rapidly expanded, so too has the intake of refined carbs and sugars. In fact, we are consuming about 22 percent more calories than we did just 30 years ago and most of them—85 percent—are from the Great White Hazards, especially sugary foods and beverages. I have no doubt that America's refined carb overload is indeed a prominent driver of our explosive obesity epidemic.

(Continued on page 44)

The Acquittal Of Carrots And Watermelon

If you have been following the recent diet wars, you may have noticed that carrots and watermelon have gotten a bad rap. However, the verdict is in and these foods have been exonerated of all their "glycemic crimes."

When researchers initially calculated the glycemic index ranking, it was based on how fast 50 carbohydrate grams of each food raised blood sugar levels. More recently, another factor called the glycemic load (GL) was added to the mix. The GL takes both the glycemic index and the average number of carbohydrate grams per serving into account. When it comes to certain foods, the glycemic load is a far more accurate measure.

Here's how it works. Carrots have a relatively high glycemic index for a vegetable, based on how fast it takes for the 50 carbohydrate grams of carrots to raise blood sugar levels. One carrot, however, has only four grams of carbohydrates; you would have to eat a pound and a half of carrots to get 50 carb grams worth! Needless to say, few people are going to eat that many carrots. To counter these contradictions, researchers now multiply the number of carbohydrate grams in a serving times the glycemic index; the resulting number is the glycemic load. Clearly, the GL of carrots puts them into an acceptable range. I eat carrots daily!

What about watermelon? Although it ranks 72 on the glycemic index, there's very little non-water substance in watermelon. If you eat a 120-gram serving (about 4.2 ounces) of watermelon, you're getting about six grams of carbs, giving it a very low glycemic load of about four. And watermelon is a great source of the powerful antioxidant lycopene—so enjoy.

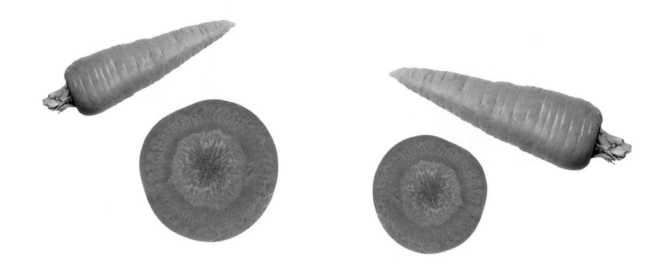

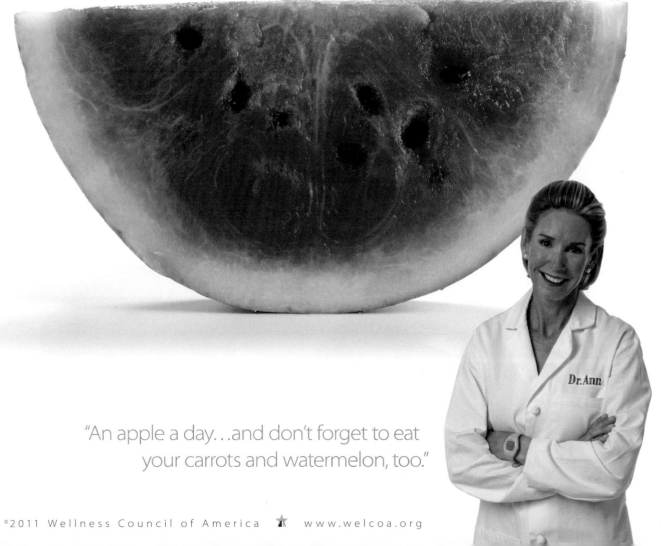

"An apple a day…and don't forget to eat your carrots and watermelon, too."

Don't
Forget!

The Great White Hazards lead to weight gain by:

1. Throwing the body into fat-storage mode.

2. Driving down blood sugar levels quickly and stimulating appetite.

Anyone who is overweight, inactive or suffers from type 2 diabetes or metabolic syndrome is most susceptible to this vicious cycle.

Now, one of insulin's most important roles is to escort glucose out of the bloodstream and deliver it to cells, where it can be used or stored for energy. If large amounts of insulin are suddenly dumped into the bloodstream, you will shortly thereafter have large amounts of glucose suddenly leaving. Excessive insulin entering the bloodstream translates to excessive glucose leaving the bloodstream and ultimately a rapid drop in blood sugar levels. In summary:

Eat the Great White Hazards ➡ blood glucose spikes ➡ blood insulin spikes ➡ blood glucose plummets

Unfortunately, the fallout from a sudden dive in blood glucose levels is none other than HUNGER. This precarious situation ultimately rings the dinner bell in your brain! We are hard-wired to despise rapidly falling blood sugar levels, as our brains are completely dependent on glucose to function. Your brain makes up about two percent of your total body weight, yet it utilizes up to 20 percent of the glucose that enters the bloodstream. So when your brain senses that blood glucose is plummeting, as a protective mechanism the appetite center housed within it immediately gets turned on. Once the brain's appetite center is activated, you experience hunger and are driven to eat. A simple way of saying all of this is that the Great White Hazards perpetuate and promote your appetite. To make matters even worse—the foods we typically desire when our blood sugar levels fall quickly are more of the Great White Hazards.

Simply put, the more you eat the Great White Hazards, the more you crave them and the more you eat them and so on. This is a critical point because the battle with body weight can often be fought and won by simply avoiding the foods that make you hungry and substituting them with the foods that make you feel full.

Understanding The
Glycemic Index
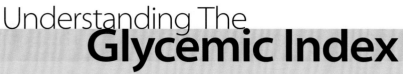

If you want to lose weight or maintain your weight, you must make an effort to eliminate or at least limit the bad carbohydrates. The glycemic index is a great tool that can help you do just this.

The glycemic index measures how various foods affect your blood sugar level. Foods are ranked on a scale from 0 to 100, according to the extent that they will raise blood sugar levels. Foods that are quickly digested or rapidly converted into sugar have a high number, while foods that are slowly digested have a low number. Here are some popular foods along with their ranking on the glycemic index:

Food	Index
Baked potato	95
White bread	95
Honey	90
Bagel	72
Milk Chocolate bar	70
Corn	70
White rice	70
Bananas	60
Jam	55
Oatmeal	55
Brown rice	50
Peas	50
Carrots	49
Whole grain pasta	40
Strawberries	40
Apples	38
Lentils/dried beans	30
Cherries	22
Soybeans	18
Broccoli	15
Tomatoes	15
Mushrooms	15

It's pretty clear that the white carbs and sweetest foods are at the top. To Eat Right For Life™, you must eat carbohydrates with a low to moderate glycemic index ranking—the right carbs. Your system will digest these carbs more slowly, thereby ensuring that your energy and blood sugar levels remain steady. Furthermore, foods with a lower ranking will not flood your system with insulin, so the cycle of blood sugar peaks and valleys will not occur.

It's impractical and unnecessary to memorize the glycemic index number of each and every food you eat. Just know that the Great White Hazards all have a high glycemic index ranking, and that the right carbs—beans, whole grains, non-starchy vegetables and fruits—largely have a low to moderate glycemic index number.

Sugar's Aliases

Here is the lowdown on the names you will see on ingredient lists that indicate sugar is added. All of these sweeteners are sugar as far as your body is concerned and will spike your blood levels of glucose and/or fructose.

- Table sugar
- Honey
- Fruit juice concentrate, ex: apple juice or grape juice concentrate
- Maple syrup
- Molasses
- Raw sugar
- Crystalline fructose
- Agave syrup or nectar
- Brown sugar
- High-fructose corn syrup (HFCS)
- Dextrose
- Corn syrup
- Evaporated cane juice

Now, the American Heart Association recommends that added sugars make up no more than 100 calories a day for women and 150 calories a day for men. I concur!

White Sugars: Not A Sweet Deal For The Body

Sugar and sugary foods and beverages are even more fattening and unhealthy than their Great White Hazard relatives (white flour, white rice, white potatoes). The sugar in foods and beverages can bypass the digestive process all together and zip straight into the bloodstream. But it gets even worse. When you eat or drink sugary products, you experience a quick surge of blood glucose *and* a surge of blood fructose. Before I go further, I want to make sure you know that all "sugars" and sugar-based sweeteners are made up of various combinations of the two simple sugars: glucose and fructose. For example, table sugar is equal parts glucose and fructose. High-fructose corn syrup is 55 percent fructose and 45 percent glucose. The rapid increase in blood fructose that ensues after consuming sweet foods and beverages is perhaps one of the most frightening and metabolically novel occurrences our bodies can experience. Over the past 20 years there has been a dramatic increase in the consumption of dietary fructose (mainly from high-fructose corn syrup and other sweeteners). It currently makes up about 15 percent of all the calories consumed in America!

Metabolically, fructose is a highly unique molecule. For starters, we know that fructose blocks the oxidation (burning) of fat in the peripheral areas of the body. But the really scary thing about fructose is what it does in the liver. When we consume fructose, it's immediately delivered to the liver because our cells are not capable of using it. However, the liver can convert fructose into a usable form of metabolic currency—either glucose or fat. The problem is that when fructose hits the liver, especially in large amounts (think a can of soda or a bowl of fruit loops) it becomes a potent stimulator of liver fat production. This metabolic property of fructose is highly significant because the buildup of fat in the liver (even very small amounts) appears to be the defining step in the development of insulin resistance. This is highly significant because insulin resistance is arguably killing more people in this country than anything else. Having insulin resistance (which currently affects 40 to 50 percent of the adult population and a growing number of kids) increases the risk of heart attacks, high blood pressure, type 2 diabetes and cancer death. It also makes it very easy to gain weight and accelerates the aging process.

New research has also recently documented that this stealth, yet tenacious fat builder prompts our desire for food. Unlike glucose, the metabolism of fructose in the brain produces by-products that directly arouse and stimulate appetite. To make matters even worse, high intakes of fructose can impair the hormone leptin. Leptin is produced by the body's fat cells and is one of the body's most powerful appetite suppressive hormones. To maintain a healthy body weight, leptin must work properly.

As you can see, there are many powerful ways that fructose can readily cause weight gain. Restricting your intake of fructose-rich foods and beverages is paramount if you want to avoid unhealthy weight gain and stay healthy. In addition to obesity and weight gain, dietary fructose has been associated with metabolic syndrome, type 2 diabetes, kidney disease, gout, high triglycerides and fatty liver disease. The greatest dietary sources of fructose are sodas, fruit drinks, sweets/desserts and sugary cereals. For optimal health, experts recommend that fructose comprise no more than three percent of your total daily calories. To achieve this, you really need to avoid or restrict the aforementioned foods and beverages. Just as with the other Great White Hazards, those who are overweight and/or inactive need to be especially vigilant in staying away from fructose-rich foods and beverages. Studies show that the adverse metabolic consequences from consuming fructose are exacerbated in those who are overweight.

Insulin Resistance: What It Is And Why You Don't Want It

I have referenced insulin resistance many times and I think it's time that I fully educate you about this growing health issue that is so needlessly robbing people of their energy and good health.

In your body, insulin functions as the "CEO" of fuel management. At the cellular level, it is insulin that's responsible for the storage of fuel, the partitioning of fuel, and the use of fuel to produce energy. When insulin becomes impaired, we define the condition that develops as insulin resistance.

Insulin resistance turns the body into a metabolic train wreck, interfering with all aspects of fuel storage and energy production. Fat cells turn into fat magnets, which makes it very easy to gain weight and difficult to lose it. Excess fuel (glucose and fat) builds up in the blood stream and cannot get into the cells that need it. This makes you tired and leads to higher blood glucose and blood fat (triglyceride) levels. Lastly, fat gets deposited in places that it normally shouldn't like your muscles, liver and heart. The fat cells that accumulate in these areas are highly unique and dangerous. They essentially spew out nasty chemicals called adipokines. Adipokines are potent, pro-inflammatory

Sweet News About
Dark Chocolate

This delectable, truly healthy treat has been shown to boost brain power, elevate mood and improve cardiovascular health. Intriguing research shows that dark chocolate may provide a greater feeling of satisfaction and satiety than other sweets. Researchers speculate that dark chocolate's potent "bittersweet" taste conveys stronger and more robust signals from the taste buds in the mouth to the satiety center of the brain. For many, this same intense flavor also means that less chocolate can do the trick. Additionally, the bit of fat in dark chocolate provides quick appetite suppression and can also hinder the absorption of its sugar, blunting those hunger-promoting spikes of blood glucose sweets typically generate.

For the healthy icing on the cake, dark chocolate may even trick your body into burning more fat. The active ingredients in dark chocolate are a class of super-potent antioxidants called flavanols. Flavanols have been shown to enhance the action of insulin and boost metabolism. They also have heart-protective benefits when eaten in moderation.

So make dark chocolate your sweet of choice! Here's my advice for doing so in a healthy and responsible way:

- Limit your indulgence to a prudent portion; no more than one ounce daily.

- Aim for high cacao content—60% or higher is optimal. The higher its percentage of cacao, the more beneficial flavanols it contains and the less sugar it provides.

Do I Have Insulin
Resistance?

Only your doctor can confirm whether or not you have insulin resistance, but here are several reliable markers that signify its presence:

- High blood pressure
- High triglycerides
- Low HDL (good) cholesterol
- A waist size greater than 35 inches in females and 40 inches in males
- Tendency to gain weight in the mid-section
- Elevated blood glucose
- Difficulty losing weight
- Lack of energy/fatigue

Remember that the Great White Hazards, especially beverages and sweets that are fructose-rich and sugary, are particularly damaging foods for those who have insulin resistance.

substances that ignite a fire of dangerous inflammation throughout the body. Scientists now believe that adipokines released from the unnatural fat that builds up in the liver, muscles and around the heart explain the direct relationship between overweight/obesity and disease. Adipokines essentially drive the development of our biggest killers: high blood pressure, abnormal blood lipid levels, type 2 diabetes and heart disease. What's especially scary is that adipokines directly impair insulin activity. This means that insulin resistance progresses further which perpetuates the whole cycle like this:

Insulin resistance ➡ unnatural fat builds up ➡ adipokines ➡ more insulin resistance ➡ more unnatural fat builds up and so on

This can become a truly deadly vicious cycle.

As previously mentioned, insulin resistance is currently an epidemic in America, affecting 40 plus percent of the adult population and a growing number of children. There are a host of behaviors that lead to insulin resistance, including gaining excess weight (especially within the belly and chest), not getting enough physical activity, and eating an unhealthy diet. Genetic factors can also contribute, but in America most people have it because of dietary and lifestyle choices. The good news is that avoiding or reversing insulin resistance is almost completely under your personal control. There are numerous things you can do to prevent insulin resistance. And if you currently have it, these very same strategies can help reverse it. The dietary prescription for the prevention and reversal of insulin resistance is provided in its entirety within this book. If you follow my *Eat Right For Life*™ plan, you will be adhering to all of the nutritional strategies that science has shown can prevent and reverse insulin resistance.

66Insulin resistance turns the body into a metabolic train wreck, interfering with all aspects of fuel storage and energy production. Fat cells turn into fat magnets, which makes it very easy to gain weight and difficult to lose it.99

The Link Between Bad Carbs And Disease

Restricting the Great White Hazards is not just about body weight—your good health also depends on it. Too much glucose, fructose and insulin pumping through your arteries not only promotes weight gain, but it can also have devastating effects on your health. People who eat the most Great White Hazards seem to more easily develop heart disease, type 2 diabetes and even cancer. The following takes a look at just how closely these bad carbs are linked to these potentially deadly diseases.

HEART DISEASE

Excess glucose and insulin are toxic to the cells that line our arteries. These cells are called endothelial cells, and they maintain the smooth and continuous blood flow so vital for life. Having too much glucose and insulin in the bloodstream interferes with the function of these important endothelial cells, and can increase blood pressure and make your blood more likely to clot. High levels of glucose and insulin also incite inflammation and promote the buildup of plaque. The Great White Hazards also have a tendency to increase blood triglycerides (a bad blood fat) while lowering good cholesterol (HDL) levels.

The literature clearly demonstrates the ill effects refined carbs have on heart health. For example, a study that followed over 75,000 adult women for a period of 10 years found that those consuming the highest glycemic diets were twice as likely to get cardiovascular disease versus those who ate the lowest glycemic diets. Women in this study who were overweight showed the strongest associations between eating refined carbs and getting heart disease. In a second study that included almost two million adults, those consuming the highest glycemic diets were 25 percent more likely to develop cardiovascular disease than those with the lowest glycemic diets. Again, keep in mind that the Great White Hazards are the worst for those who are already overweight or obese, but ultimately everyone should stay away from these foods.

TYPE 2 DIABETES

There has been an explosion in the occurrence of type 2 diabetes over the last two decades and it remains America's fastest growing epidemic—affecting about 12 percent of the population. Risk factors for this deadly disease include:

- Overweight/obesity (especially abdominal obesity)
- Physical inactivity
- Family history
- An unhealthy diet

If you have any of these traits, it is imperative that you restrict the Great White Hazards to maintain your health and vitality.

Results from the highly esteemed Harvard-based Nurses' Health Study confirm refined carbs are the foods eaten most commonly by people who develop type 2 diabetes. A study performed by a group of Australian

Don't Let Yourself Get Hungry

It takes fewer calories to prevent hunger than it does to deal with it once it occurs. Be sure to include three meals a day, along with a mid-afternoon snack to avoid ravenous hunger. Regularly including breakfast with a nice dose of protein is particularly valuable for reining in appetite, so do not skip this morning feeding. My top rated mid-afternoon snack is a handful of nuts. Other excellent snack choices include:

- Pumpkin seeds or sunflower seeds
- Cut fresh veggies (carrots, celery, bell peppers, broccoli, cauliflower etc.)—dip in hummus/bean dips, guacamole, salsa, or olive oil and vinegar.
- Fresh or frozen fruit
- Soy nuts, dried wasabi peas
- 100% whole grain crackers like AK-mak, Triscuits or pita chips with reduced-fat cheese, peanut butter, hummus, salsa, guacamole, sardines or smoked salmon
- Stone ground tortilla chips (I love "Food Should Taste Good' brand) dipped in hummus, salsa or guacamole
- Low-fat plain yogurt with some fresh cut up fruit
- Part-skim mozzarella or other reduced-fat (2% milk) cheeses (try convenient cheese sticks)
- Homemade fruit smoothies with some ground hemp seed powder
- Trail mix (avoid dried fruit if overweight, diabetic or insulin resistant)
- Dried whole grain cereals
- Granola bars (Kashi is my favorite brand)
- Hard-boiled omega-3 eggs
- Dark chocolate—60% or more cacao—in moderation!

How To Curb Your
Cravings

I am frequently asked, "How can I overcome my cravings for white breads and sugars?" Here is my best advice:

1. **Consciously recognize sugar cravings** as a convenient reminder of how important it is to eat a healthy diet.

2. **Restrict the foods that precipitously drop your blood sugar.** Namely, the Great White Hazards— white flour products, white rice, white potatoes and sugar/sweets. Sugar cravings are a good indicator that you are consuming too many Great White Hazards.

3. **Eat three meals daily** with a mid-afternoon snack to avoid over-indulgence later in the day. Deprivation or marked hunger can increase cravings for sweet foods. It's especially important to eat breakfast, as skipping breakfast has been associated with increased food cravings.

4. **Have a healthy protein at each meal.** Protein provides a stable and more prolonged blood sugar level.

5. **Regularly include the "slower carbs"**—whole grains, beans, fruits and non-starchy veggies.

(Continued on following page)

investigators followed 36,787 adults over a four-year period, and found those who ate the most white bread were 30 percent more likely to develop type 2 diabetes. Finally, a systematic review of 37 prior studies found that those who consumed the highest glycemic diets were 40 percent more likely to develop type 2 diabetes than those consuming the lowest glycemic diets.

The underlying metabolic problem in type 2 diabetes is largely insulin resistance. Victims of type 2 diabetes typically suffer some degree of insulin resistance for many years prior to fully developing the disease. If your insulin doesn't work well and you eat the Great White Hazards, your pancreas has to work extra hard and is forced to release more insulin to get all of the blood sugar into your cells. Repeating this scenario over time eventually outstrips the supply of insulin the pancreas is capable of producing. As a result, you develop insufficient blood insulin levels, and your cells are not able to absorb the blood glucose they need to survive. Blood glucose levels then rise abnormally high, signifying the development of full-blown type 2 diabetes.

CANCER

The defining feature of all cancers is uncontrolled cellular growth. Anything that promotes cellular growth in the body can increase the likelihood that a cell will become cancerous. Consuming the Great White Hazards may just be such a factor. In fact, many studies have shown a link between America's "typical western diet" and some of the most life-threatening cancers. Of course, the westernized diet is often high in refined, high glycemic carbohydrates. Although the exact relationship between eating lots of refined carbs and increasing your cancer risk has not been fully elucidated, many scientists speculate the answer lies with the high blood insulin levels refined carb diets generate. The hormone insulin is a trigger for the release of a second hormone called insulin-like-growth-factor-1 (IGF-1). Both insulin and IGF-1 stimulate cells to divide while simultaneously blocking cell death (a very bad combination in terms of cancer risk).

Laboratory studies have specifically shown that cells of the prostate, colon and breast respond to insulin-like-growth-factor-1. High blood insulin levels can lead to excessive IGF-1 production. Too much IGF-1 may lead to excessive cellular proliferation in these tissues, and ultimately to cancer itself. A study published in the *Journal of the National Cancer Institute* reported that women who consumed the highest glycemic diets were nearly three times more likely to develop colon cancer compared to women with the lowest glycemic diets.

Another scientific finding suggests that elevated blood insulin levels promote cancer. This study was published in the *New England Journal of Medicine* and found that overweight/obesity accounts for 20 percent of cancer deaths in women and 14 percent of cancer deaths in men. That is a total of 90,000 U.S. cancer deaths annually attributed solely to being overweight. Investigators hypothesize that an elevated blood insulin level, common in those with excess body fat, may very well be one of the reasons for their observations.

It's Time To Break Up With The Bad Carbs

No matter how much you love your white carbs and sweets, you need to curtail and limit your intake of them. Simply put, if you don't restrict or eliminate the Great White Hazards, losing or maintaining weight will almost be insurmountable. Believe me, once you cut these foods from your diet, you will barely miss them. Instead of craving the wrong carbs like baked potatoes, a big hunk of white bread or a bottle of soda, you will begin to crave the right carbs like beans, whole grains, non-starchy vegetables and fruits. And just wait—once you feel and experience what the right carbs can do for your health, energy level and physique, you will be hooked for life.

The Right Carbs

When it comes to maximizing your state of wellness and increasing your chances of successful and permanent weight loss, learning how to do your carbs right is one of the most powerful nutritional strategies you can incorporate into your daily life. Now that we have tackled the wrong carbs, we can start discussing the four delicious categories of right carbs: whole grains, beans, vegetables and fruits. These carbohydrates contain a bounty of health-promoting agents including vitamins, minerals, fiber and those amazing, disease-busting phytochemicals. Plus, unlike the Great White Hazards, they are digested slowly, resulting in a more gradual and gentle blood glucose and insulin response.

We will discuss veggies and fruit at length in the following section, so at the moment, I want to introduce you to the two other right carbs: beans and grains. Replacing the Great White Hazards with these good carbs provides an enormous opportunity to safeguard your health. Relish these good-for-you foods because they can lower your risk of heart disease, improve your gastrointestinal health, lower your risk of many cancers, protect against type 2 diabetes, and help you lose weight!

The Wonderful Benefits Of Beans

I consider beans the most underutilized economical super food. Beans, along with peas and lentils, are members of the legume family of vegetables. They are all versatile, convenient, cheap, tasty, satisfying and remarkably good for you. Indeed, beans have megawatt nutritional power. Beans are an outstanding source of several key minerals including iron, magnesium, calcium and potassium. They provide the full family of B vitamins, including more folate than any other food. Folate is the B vitamin famous for its heart-healthy and cancer protective properties.

(Continued on page 54)

How To Curb Your Cravings

(Continued from previous page)

6. **Avoid artificially sweetened foods and beverages.** Artificial sweeteners are exquisitely sweet substances that exploit our highly developed taste for sweets and keep our taste buds in overdrive. The good news is that you can easily train your tastes. In other words, the less sweet foods you eat, the sweeter they taste when you have them—and vice versa.

7. **Recognize that there are healthier ways to satisfy your sweet tooth** and keep these alternatives conveniently on hand:

➤ Dark chocolate (60% or more cacao)—my top rated sweet

➤ 100% fruit sorbets, sherbets and/or low-fat yogurt

➤ 100% frozen fruit bars

➤ Granola bars

➤ Dried fruit (apricots, raisins, prunes, apples, etc.) You can even freeze them, which gives them a gummy bear-like consistency

➤ Fresh fruit topped with low-fat plain yogurt blended with a little maple syrup

➤ Hot chocolate made from skim milk and 100% real cocoa powder

➤ Sweetened 100% whole grain cereals. Choose those with 10 grams or less of sugar per serving.

It's very simple to identify the bad carbs because they are all white. This notorious group of carbs includes white flour products, white rice, white potatoes and sugar. Scientifically, they are known as the highly refined, high glycemic carbs. However, I refer to them as the "Great White Hazards."

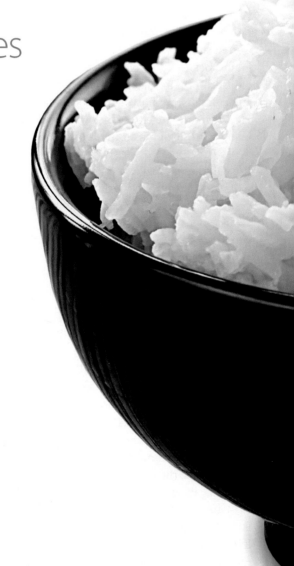

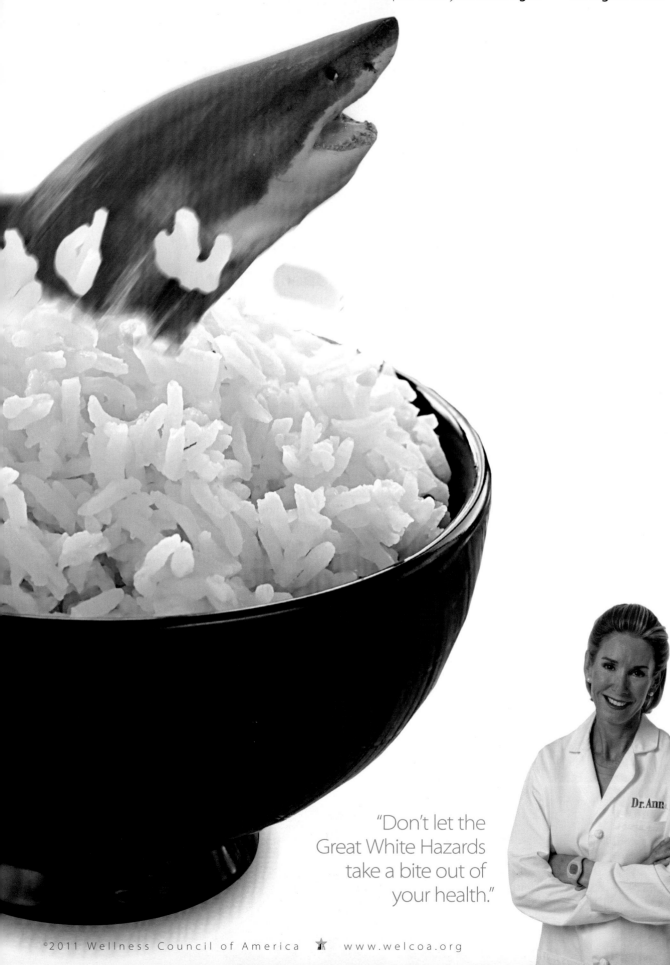

"Don't let the Great White Hazards take a bite out of your health."

The Side Effect Of
Beans

Some people suffer from gas when they eat beans. When your digestive enzymes are unable to break down all of the starch contained in beans, the bacteria in your colon will often ferment the remnants. Gas is a natural by-product of this fermentation process. If you are one of the unfortunate individuals who experience this uncomfortable (and occasionally embarrassing) situation, try these gas-troubleshooting tips:

- Consume the beans/legumes known to cause the least amount of gas—lima beans, anasazi, black eyed peas, chick peas, mung beans, split peas and lentils.

- Discard the cooking liquid and rinse beans in fresh water before consuming them.

- Rinse canned beans thoroughly.

- Don't consume a large quantity of beans in one sitting.

- Use a pressure cooker.

- Cook your beans with a little ginger, fennel or anise—all are natural gas-reducers.

- Consider using Beano or another over-the-counter digestive enzyme product.

The Greatest Source Of Fiber

Beans are chock full of fiber, providing more than any other food. A single cup of beans provides a whopping 12 grams of fiber. This single serving is the amount of fiber the average American gets in an entire day! Beans are especially high in soluble fiber, a type of fiber that has powerful cholesterol-lowering effects. Beans' soluble fiber also makes them especially useful for those with insulin resistance and type 2 diabetes. Soluble fiber forms a gelatinous mass within the gastrointestinal tract that slows the absorption of glucose into the bloodstream. This helps keep blood sugar levels lower and steadier. Beans also provide a nice dose of insoluble fiber. This is the kind of fiber that promotes regularity and prevents digestive problems like diverticulitis.

Unparalleled Appetite Control

Beans are unmatched in their ability to control appetite and body weight. With their unique high protein, high fiber make up, beans can fill you up without filling you out. Moreover, beans have more protein than any other plant food, and protein is nature's diet pill—giving rise to longer lasting appetite suppression than any other macronutrient. Beans' hefty dose of zero calorie, yet "filling" fiber plays a starring role in appetite control too. Even with their starchy makeup, beans will not increase your blood sugar levels. To the contrary, with the exception of non-starchy vegetables, beans have a lower glycemic response than any of the right carbs.

An All-Around Super Food

Like other plant foods, beans are also teeming with antioxidant phytochemicals, including flavanoids. Of the foods with the most antioxidant power, four different beans make it into the top 20 list. Beans' stellar nutritional profile and rich supply of antioxidants qualify them as true health champions. It is no wonder that people who eat more beans tend to be leaner, get less heart disease, high blood pressure, type 2 diabetes, and colon and breast cancer.

A study including nearly 10,000 U.S. adults found that those who consumed beans four or more times a week were 22 percent less likely to get heart disease than those who had them less than once a week. A second study involving over 64,000 Asian women found that those consuming the most legumes, including soybeans, were 38 percent less likely to develop type 2 diabetes.

Canned, fresh, frozen or dried—all beans are great for you. Enjoy all beans any way you want: Bean dips, bean soups, beans in your salads, beans in your whole grain burritos, beans in your stews, beans in your rice, beans in your chili, beans in your stir-fry—just eat more beans!

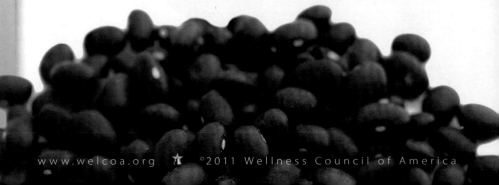

The Greatness Of Whole Grains

Let's move on to the second group of healthy, right carbs—whole grains. True whole grains are among the most powerful, disease-fighting foods nature has given us. Unlike their refined, Great White Hazard counterparts, whole grains retain all of their dazzling nutritional goodness. When whole grains are refined and processed into products like white flour and white rice, their outer bran coat and their inner germ portions are removed. Unfortunately, these are the two areas that house virtually all of a whole grain's nutritional power. So a refined grain is nothing more than a whole grain with all of its nutritional goodness removed. This is an especially disheartening reality given that the average American eats more than five servings of refined grains and less than one serving of whole grains a day. In fact, only seven percent of Americans are eating the daily recommendation of three or more servings of whole grains.

Whole grains are a virtual treasure trove of nutrients. They are excellent sources of vitamin E, B vitamins, fiber, and the minerals zinc, iron and magnesium. Like other plant-based foods, they are abundant in health-boosting phytochemicals, including polyphenols and phytoestrogens. They contain cholesterol-lowering phytosterols and an abundance of gut-friendly insoluble fiber. In summary, whole grains offer a unique and powerful constellation of nutritional attributes.

People who eat the most whole grains weigh less, and are less likely to develop heart disease, type 2 diabetes, cancers, metabolic syndrome and digestive diseases. When it comes to studies on whole grains and health, whole grains are rapidly approaching fruits and vegetables as nature's most life-preserving foods.

Great For Disease Protection

A review of seven major investigations found that study subjects who consumed just 2.5 servings of whole grains daily reduced their risk of cardiovascular disease by 25 percent. The Nurses' Health Study found that non-smokers who ate three servings of whole grains a day were 50 percent less likely to get heart disease than those who rarely ate whole grains. Another study found that those consuming the most whole grains had lower BMI's (body mass index), smaller waists, lower cholesterol levels and healthier blood glucose levels. A review of 40 different studies evaluating the impact of whole grains on cancer risk found that including as little as three or four servings of whole grains weekly can provide protection from many different forms of cancer.

©2011 Wellness Council of America ★ www.welcoa.org

Whole Grains Have Lots Of
Antioxidants Too!

In a first-of-its-kind evaluation, scientists found that many of the popular whole grain breakfast cereals and even whole grain snack foods provide "surprisingly large" amounts of antioxidant polyphenols—gram for gram, levels on par with those in fruits and veggies! Of the whole grain snack foods tested, popcorn came out on top. For cereals, those made from wheat were the antioxidant winners followed by corn, oats and then rice. (*Journal of Agricultural and food Chemistry*, July 2009).

Choosing A Healthy
Cereal

Cereals offer a tasty and convenient way to get in your whole grains. Yet, not all cereals are created equal. In fact, some cereals have more sugar per serving than soda! Here are two simple rules to help you make a healthy and wholesome choice. Check the cereal's nutrition facts box.

- Make sure the cereal contains five grams or more of fiber per serving.

- Be sure it contains 10 grams or less of sugar per serving.

Thankfully, there are upwards of 30 different varieties of cereal available that fit this bill.

Switch Out The Bad For
The Good

I want everybody to replace the Great White Hazards with the right carbs, and a powerful report published in the *American Journal of Clinical Nutrition* beautifully sums up why this is so important. The report comprised the most definitive review to date of the impact sugar and refined carbs have on disease risk. In this combined analysis of 37 forward-looking studies, scientists found that high glycemic diets "independently increased the risk of type 2 diabetes, heart disease, gall bladder disease, breast cancer, and all diseases combined." A key finding of this evaluation was that diets heavy in sugar and refined carbs are demonstrably bad for you. In fact, removing these foods from your diet provides the same or even more health protection than simply including more whole grains and fiber in your diet.

To give you perspective, regularly eating whole grains provides a 20 to 40 percent reduction in heart disease and a 20 to 30 percent reduction in type 2 diabetes versus sparse consumption. You can potentially more than double that protection by simply replacing products high in sugar and refined carbs with whole grains. That's now easier than ever to do!

Great For The Waistline

In stark contrast to the Great White Hazards, whole grains can help you achieve and maintain a healthy body weight. Because whole grains retain all of their natural fiber and have not been processed, they are more difficult to digest. Your system has to work longer and harder to break down and absorb their starch (glucose). This means that whole grains, especially physically intact varieties like oats and brown rice, have a much lower and more favorable glycemic response. Additionally, scientists believe whole grains' abundance of magnesium, antioxidants and plant fibers facilitate insulin's action, which helps keep your metabolism running smoothly and effectively. The Nurses' Health Study found that women who ate the most fiber-rich whole grains gained significantly less weight over time than those getting the least.

Great Tasting

There are many different varieties of great tasting whole grains to choose from, including traditional American favorites like oatmeal and whole wheat bread to exotic grains like quinoa and triticale. When you are selecting your whole grain foods, always be sure they are 100 percent whole grain varieties. Look for "100 percent whole grain" or "100 percent whole wheat" on the label. Just note that labeling laws can be very tricky with whole grain products. If "most" (i.e. 51 percent or more) of the grain in the product is whole, it can be labeled "whole grain" or "whole wheat" (but you will not see "100 percent"). Look for "100 percent" on the label and double check for the word "whole" listed before any grain in the ingredients list. If you see "wheat flour," "enriched wheat flour" or any other grain listed without the word "whole" in front of it, it's nothing more than refined flour disguised as the healthier option.

Choose what you enjoy, but strive for physically intact grains and dense high fiber cereals as your first choices. Although 100 percent whole grain or 100 percent whole wheat breads are good carb choices, the physical processing that occurs in these products means they are much easier to digest and can bump up blood glucose more readily than intact whole grains. For this reason, I prefer you choose oatmeal, barley, quinoa, bulgur, brown rice and high fiber cereals over whole grain or whole wheat breads. For those who have insulin resistance, (diabetics, pre-diabetics and those with metabolic syndrome) I recommend you forgo all bread and bread products completely and simply stick to physically intact grains and dense high fiber (five grams or more per serving) cereals. For optimal health, everyone should include three servings or more of 100 percent whole grains (preferably physically intact varieties) daily. A serving includes ½ cup cooked whole grains, a single slice of bread, or ¼ to ¾ cups of prepared breakfast cereals (check the cereal box nutrition label for specifics).

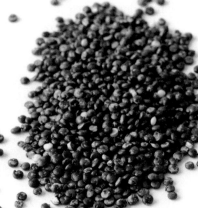

Use the following *Do Your Carbs Right Plan Of Action* to guide you in replacing the wrong carbs with the right ones.

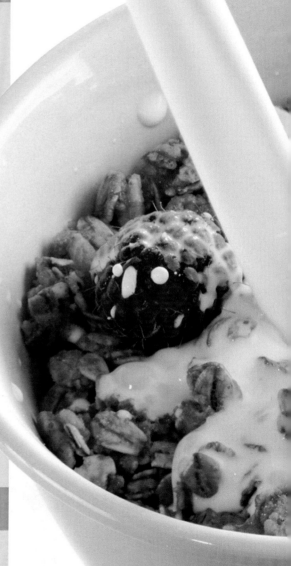

PLAN OF ACTION — Do your carbs **right.**

1. MINIMIZE THE GREAT WHITE HAZARDS

These quickly digested, high glycemic carbs spike your blood glucose and insulin levels, which promotes weight gain, cardiovascular disease, type 2 diabetes, certain cancers and macular degeneration. Sugar and sugary foods and beverages also spike your blood fructose levels.

- Avoid foods made from white flour. This includes white breads, cakes, cookies, pasta, pastries, bagels, biscuits, rolls, crackers, pancakes, waffles, dumplings, sugary junk cereals, pretzels and pizza dough. Choose 100 percent whole grain or multigrain varieties instead. If you love pasta, the multigrain varieties like Barilla Plus taste like regular pasta and are acceptable.

- Avoid white rice—Choose brown rice instead. Brown rice is a physically intact whole grain. If white rice is a must, then converted or basmati brands are a healthier choice as they have a more favorable glycemic response.

- Avoid white potatoes in any form—baked, mashed, French fried or boiled—Small, new potatoes with skin are acceptable in moderation. Sweet potatoes are fine.

- Restrict sugars and sweets—Choose a prudent portion of high quality dark chocolate (60 percent or higher cacao) or fresh fruit as your dessert/sweet of choice.

- Strictly avoid sugary beverages—soda, fruit drinks, dessert coffees, sports drinks, sweet tea and tonic water.

2. ENJOY BEANS REGULARLY

- Strive to have at least one serving (½ cup) every day.

- Any variety of beans is fantastic—black beans, edamame, kidney beans, lentils, field peas, cannellini beans, navy beans, chick peas, white beans, pinto beans, anasazi beans, crowder peas, split peas, etc.

- Any form of beans is fine—canned (low sodium best), fresh, frozen or dried.

3. ALWAYS CHOOSE 100% WHOLE GRAIN OR WHOLE WHEAT VARIETIES FOR ALL GRAIN PRODUCTS

- Look for "100 percent" on the label or package.

- Strive for three or more servings a day. A serving is ½ cup cooked whole grains like brown rice or oatmeal or a single slice of bread.

- Physically intact whole grains are the healthiest choice—oats (oatmeal), brown rice, barley, bulgur, etc..

- If you are overweight, diabetic, pre-diabetic or have metabolic syndrome, it is best to stick to physically intact grains and high-fiber cereals and avoid all flour-based or bread products (even the 100 percent whole grain ones).

[CHAPTER 3]
Eat your **fruits**

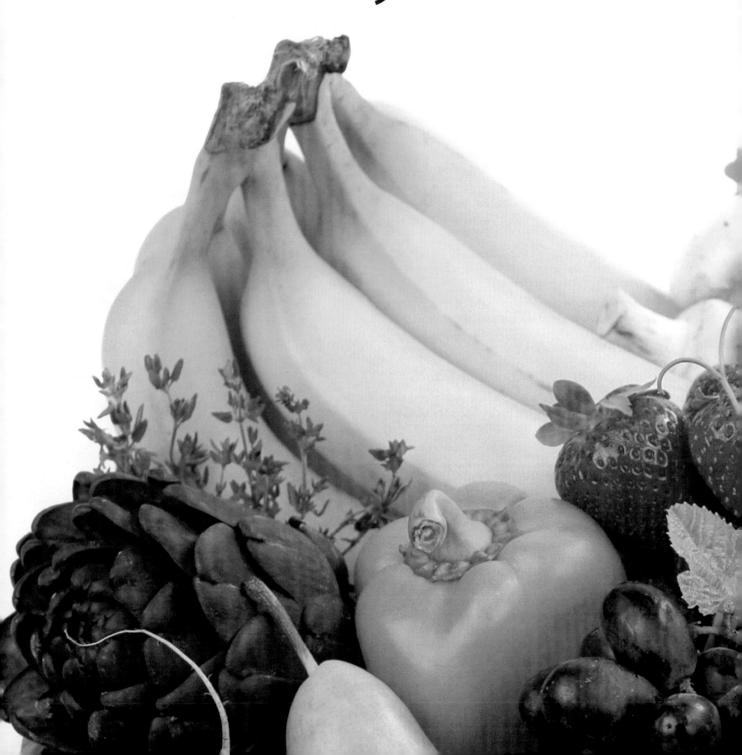

and veggies

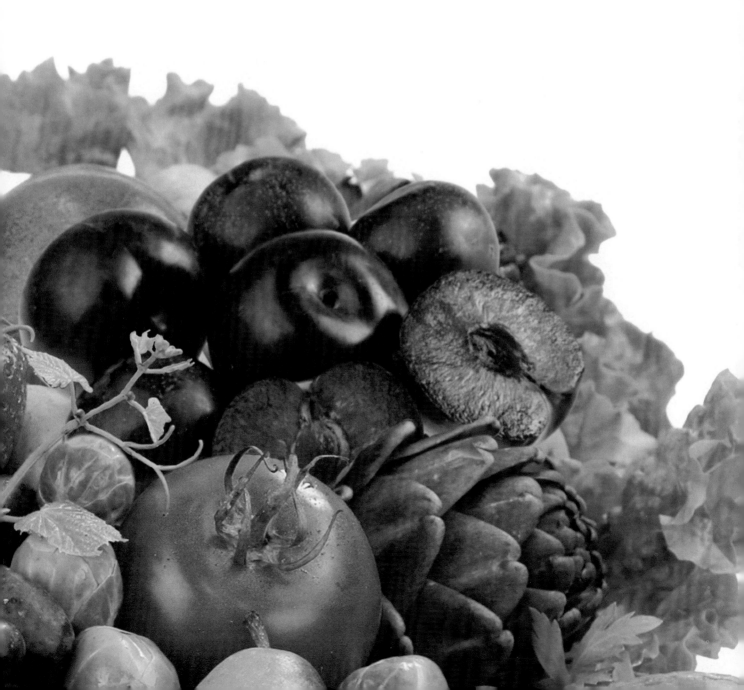

[CHAPTER 3]

Eat your fruits and veggies

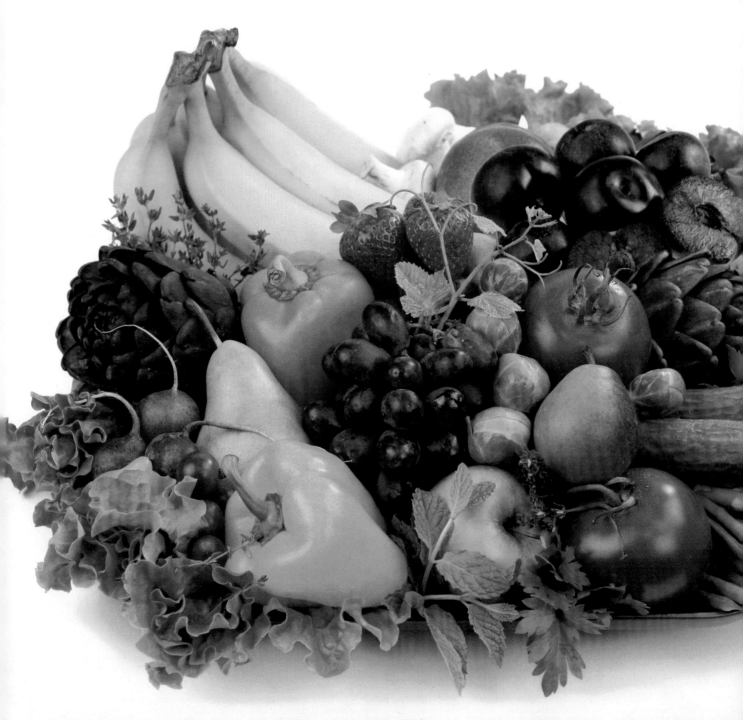

O ur journey into the wonderful world of eating right now brings us to the two remaining categories of carbs: fruits and vegetables. Fruits and vegetables are my favorite nutrition topic. Every time you include this amazing food group in your diet, you immediately improve your health. I regard fruits and vegetables so highly that I think people should be racing to their grocery stores to grab them before they're all gone!

So what exactly makes these foods so awesome? Well, for starters, fruits and vegetables are high in nutrients, yet low in calories, which is a great combo. They are bursting with an assortment of vitamins and minerals, and they offer loads of beneficial zero-calorie fiber, which means you can eat plenty without worries of weight gain. In fact, for most of us, the more fruits and vegetables we eat, the less we will weigh.

When it comes to fruits and vegetables, the first thing I want to talk about is phytochemicals. Phytochemicals are really what catapults fruits and vegetables into a league of their own. I want you to have a basic understanding of what phytochemicals are, and what they can do in your body, because I know from personal experience that it will motivate you to eat more fruit and veggies.

The Phytochemical Lowdown

The first phytochemical was just discovered about 30 years ago and I remember it vividly. Aware of my passion for nutrition and my family history of breast cancer, my father, then a practicing cancer surgeon, called to let me know scientists had discovered a breast cancer-fighting compound in broccoli. This was the very first phytochemical identified. It's called sulforaphane and it is now widely known for its cancer-fighting prowess. Since that time, more than 10,000 phytochemicals have been identified, and scientists speculate there are up to 100,000 phytochemicals yet to be discovered. You may be familiar with some phytochemicals already— lycopene found in tomatoes, resveratrol found in red wine, and flavanols found in dark chocolate. The study of phytochemicals is a very exciting area of nutritional science, as these substances offer an unmatched ability to protect our cells from damage. Drug companies can only dream of creating substances that do what phytochemicals can do with no side effects!

Plants produce phytochemicals to protect themselves against environmental elements, such as the damaging effects of the sun and plant-eating parasites. Phytochemicals essentially help plants survive and thrive. And it turns out that phytochemicals can do the same for us.

My Favorite Fruit

Berries are low in calories, high in fiber and loaded with phyto-chemicals. Here's a closer look at my favorite fruits and the wonderful benefits they provide.

Raspberries are packed with more fiber than any other fruit. They are also an outstanding source of vitamin C and manganese, and contain 10 other essential nutrients and phytochemicals, including ellagic acid (a prominent cancer-fighting substance).

Strawberries are an excellent source of vitamin C. Believe it or not, strawberries contain more vitamin C than oranges. They're also good sources of folic acid and potassium, which are two important nutrients for heart health.

Blueberries hold first place out of 49 other fruit and vegetable contenders on Tufts University's ORAC score (a measure of antioxidant power). Blueberries' anti-inflammatory power rivals their antioxidant power. This unique "one-two" punch makes blueberries the perfect brain food, as the brain is uniquely susceptible to the destructive effects of oxidation and inflammation.

Blackberries come in a close second behind blueberries in the ORAC score. They are also an excellent source of vitamin C, potassium and folate, and are rich in antioxidants, including vitamin E, ellagic acid and anthocyanin pigments.

Best of all, berries can be enjoyed in a variety of ways. Enjoy them fresh or frozen, eat them alone or toss them into salads, smoothies, yogurt, cereal or cottage cheese. Yum!

The Power Of Phytochemicals

Phytochemicals protect the human body in four primary ways. First, they offer powerful inflammation protection. In this book, I've mentioned that inflammation is a fundamental driver of many chronic diseases. However, if you consume fruits and vegetables, you can readily tap into potent anti-inflammatory phytochemicals. Phytochemicals also provide robust antioxidant power. Antioxidants neutralize toxic agents in our bodies called free radicals. Free radicals attack and damage critical areas of our cells and ultimately initiate disease and aging. Some phytochemicals comprise the most potent antioxidants ever identified. Phytochemicals also provide immune-boosting activity. The phytochemicals in fruits and veggies provide your immune system a nice turbo charge, kicking up its efficiency and effectiveness. Lastly, some phytochemicals shore up the body's innate detoxification systems. Think of them as your body's personal fleet of garbage men, working 24/7 to keep your body clear of toxic substances.

Keep in mind that these miraculous agents of good health can only be found in plant-based foods, namely fruits, vegetables, beans, whole grains, nuts and seeds. Be forewarned that you miss out on these life-preserving chemicals if you choose supplements, meal replacement bars and protein powders in lieu of eating real plant foods.

Let's now take a closer look at a few of the most famous phytochemicals.

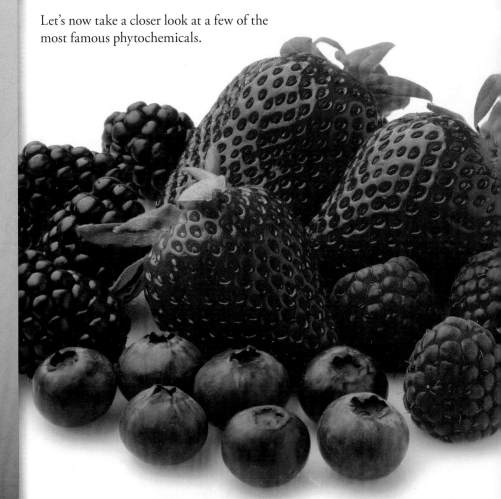

Three Phytochemicals You Need To Know About

I am certain that a brief profile of these three amazing plant chemicals will compel you to eat your fruits and vegetables with hearty and renewed enthusiasm.

LYCOPENE

Lycopene gives tomatoes their vivid red color and is one of the most potent antioxidants ever identified. As we touched on earlier, antioxidants are scavengers of rogue molecules called free radicals, which initiate a cascade of damaging oxidation. Free radicals are by-products of the body's normal metabolic processes, although they can also enter our bodies from environmental sources like tobacco smoke, smog, prescription drugs, ultraviolet radiation and even the foods we eat. The oxidation induced by free radicals damages vital cellular structures and ultimately contributes to the development of cancer, heart disease, cataracts, arthritis, and even the aging process itself. Good thing lycopene provides protection from all of these conditions!

As an anti-cancer agent, lycopene seems to protect the prostate the most zealously. A Harvard-based study published in the *Journal of the National Cancer Institute* found that men who consumed 10 or more tomato products a week reduced their risk of aggressive prostate cancer by nearly 50 percent. Furthermore, research has revealed that lycopene's protective power is enhanced when tomatoes are processed and/or cooked, so enjoy salsa, tomato paste, and marinara sauce too.

ANTHOCYANINS

Blueberries owe their deep, blue color to a class of phytochemicals called anthocyanins. Like lycopene, anthocyanins have potent antioxidant power, but they are also true workhorses when it comes to fighting inflammation. Science now tells us that excessive inflammation plays a major role in the development of several diseases, including heart attacks, some cancers, Alzheimer's, autoimmune disease, and allergic conditions. When you regularly consume blueberries, along with other anthocyanin-rich foods like cherries, blackberries and raspberries, you are protecting your body from some of the most common and deadliest illnesses known to man.

SULFORAPHANE

Broccoli is teeming with sulforaphane, one of the most powerful anti-cancer compounds nature provides. Like lycopene and anthocyanins, this phytochemical is also a potent antioxidant. Its special cancer-fighting powers are largely due to its ability to boost the body's detoxifying enzyme systems. Eating your broccoli, along with other cruciferous veggies including cabbage, kale, cauliflower, brussels sprouts and collards, will send your detoxifying, cancer-protective enzyme systems into overdrive.

(Continued on page 66)

Calling Out All Men

Fruits & Vegetables Matter

Eating an abundance of brightly colored fruits and vegetables brimming with phytochemicals is akin to adding a turbo engine to a car. Phytochemicals supercharge the body's metabolic engine so that our natural biological processes occur faster and more efficiently than they would otherwise. This is an especially apt metaphor for all of the veggie-resistant gentlemen out there—and according to the National Cancer Institute (NCI), there are quite a few of you. The NCI reports that 96 percent of the American male population does not get the recommended seven to nine servings of fruits and vegetables a day. Men are often trained to pile on the protein from an early age, and in the process, they often fail to realize that vegetables are also integral to building muscle, strength, stamina and strong bones. If you need to incorporate more fruits and vegetables into your diet, here are a few snack and meal strategies:

- Eat sliced apples with almond butter
- Toss a handful of veggies in an omelet
- Add extra lettuce, tomatoes and onions to your sandwich
- Put some dried apricots in your cereal
- Add grilled onions and mushrooms to any chicken dish

Remember, fruits and vegetables really matter, as they provide protection from the conditions men are most prone to, namely cancer and heart attacks. They also enhance physique, so load up!

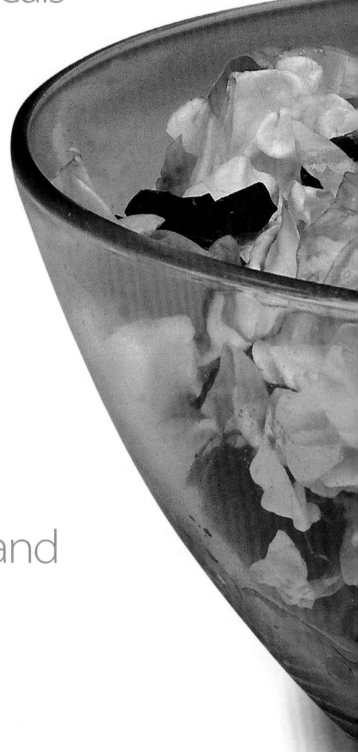

The phytochemicals in fruits and veggies provide your immune system a nice turbo charge, kicking up its efficiency and effectiveness.

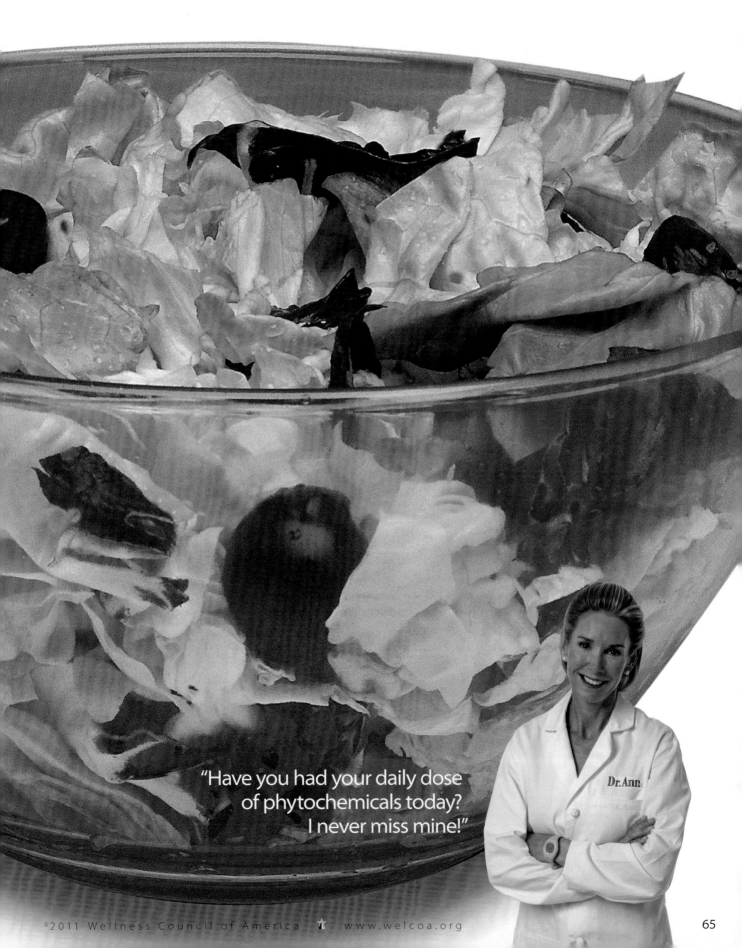

"Have you had your daily dose
of phytochemicals today?
I never miss mine!"

Did You Know You Can
"Eat" Your SPF?

Did you know that some of the same pigments that give plant foods their deep, rich color can provide "built-in" SPF for your skin? Certain phytochemicals can indeed provide valuable skin protection against the ravages of excess ultraviolet radiation (sun exposure). When you eat plant foods, some of their phytochemicals are actually deposited in your skin. The most potent SPF foods include dark leafy greens, sweet potatoes, tomatoes, carrots, red and orange bell peppers, berries, and even dark chocolate. If you include these foods in your diet regularly, your skin will develop a subtle, orange cast, (especially visible in your palms) which is visual proof of your success. To see my orange palms and to learn about other superstar foods for your skin, visit DrAnnwellness.com and watch my "Super Foods for Skin" video.

Fruits & Veggies: Our Magic Bullet

Fruits and vegetables provide powerful, broad-spectrum disease protection. Eating a diet chock-full of fruits and vegetables can help ward off heart attacks, strokes, high blood pressure, gastrointestinal diseases, Alzheimer's, cataracts, macular degeneration, type 2 diabetes as well as a host of cancers.

For optimal success, you should aim to eat as many and as much of a variety of fruits and veggies as you possibly can. When it comes to food and vitality—fruits and veggies are your magic bullet! In fact, there are thousands of scientific studies that document fruits and vegetables' ability to protect our health. Below are some of the primary diseases fruits and veggies protect us from.

Cardiovascular Disease

The famous DASH clinical trial provides perhaps some of the most favorable scientific evidence for fruits and vegetables. In this intervention study (the kind that proves cause and effect), subjects were placed on a diet rich in fruits and veggies (seven-plus servings a day) and low-fat dairy products. At the end of the eight-week trial, the study group eating the DASH diet lowered their blood pressure as effectively as standard doses of prescription blood pressure medications. Subsequent studies of the DASH diet have found it also lowers cholesterol and reduces the risk of type 2 diabetes. According to the largest and longest study to date, those who consumed the most fruits and vegetables (about eight servings a day) were 30 percent less likely to have a heart attack or stroke. Further, in a 28-year study involving more than 10,000 men and women, those consuming the most flavonoids (a large class of antioxidant phytochemicals abundant in apples, berries and onions) were less likely to die from heart attacks and strokes or develop chronic diseases, including asthma, diabetes, and lung cancer.

Cancer

Population studies have consistently linked fruit and vegetable intake to a reduced risk of cancer. According to the most definitive review of food and cancer studies, evidence is especially strong for cancers of the mouth, throat, esophagus and stomach. According to the American Institute of Cancer Research, if everyone ate the recommended amount of fruits and vegetables, 20 percent or more of all cancer cases could be prevented.

For optimal success, you should aim to eat as many and as much of a variety of fruits and veggies as you possibly can. When it comes to food and vitality— fruits and veggies are your magic bullet!

Don't Be Color-Blind!

The more colorful the food, the more it's packed with valuable nutrients. Eat from the entire spectrum to fully leverage the tens of thousands of beneficial compounds these foods offer. Have a little bit of every color: blue and purple (blueberries, eggplant, etc.), red and green (peppers, apples, spinach, etc.), and yellow (peppers, squash, bananas, etc.) each and every day. Remember, color means health: the deeper and richer the color, the more phytochemicals, vitamins and minerals present in the food. Red grapefruit is always a healthier choice than white grapefruit; red onions are better than yellow onions; deep green romaine lettuce is certainly healthier than iceberg. In fact, dark leafy greens are a nutritional Goliath, packing more nutrition per unit calorie than any other food. For perspective, consider that 100 calories of kale provides 190 times more calcium, four times more iron, 12 times more magnesium, 15 times more folate, 800 times more vitamin A, two times more protein and 11,000 times more antioxidant power than 100 calories of sirloin. Be sure to include some form of dark leafy greens in your diet each day!

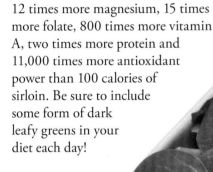

A Quick Veggie Tip

Roasted vegetables are so tasty that you won't believe you're eating "health food." This wonderful cooking technique capitalizes on the natural taste of vegetables. Virtually any vegetable can be roasted (remember to stay away from white potatoes, though). Simply place your vegetables of choice on a cookie sheet and mist them lightly with canola or olive oil pan sprays, or toss them in a little olive oil. Season them to your preference—try a little kosher salt, pepper and garlic. Roast at 375 degrees for 15 to 25 minutes or until they have a golden to brown covering and texture that suits you. Sprinkle with a little balsamic vinegar and dig in. My favorite vegetables to roast are cauliflower, sweet potatoes, brussels sprouts, carrots, and asparagus.

Weapons Of Mass
Protection

Infusing our bodies with a constant and steady stream of antioxidants should be the bedrock for healthy living. We know that oxidative stress at the cellular level is a key driver of aging and many chronic diseases. However, a recent landmark study reveals the major role antioxidants play in providing cancer protection. This study monitored genetic mutations through the human equivalent of 5,000 years and revealed that the majority of all genetic mutations (the defining step in cancer development) occur through oxidative damage. In other words, plant foods are the most powerful weapons you have for combating chronic diseases and aging. The plant foods that provide the most potent antioxidants include: red onions, tomatoes, broccoli, Brussels sprouts, red bell peppers, garlic, dark leafy greens, apples, red grapes, berries, pomegranates, cherries, oranges, plums, black beans, kidney beans, tea and dark chocolate. Go eat some now!

It's Not All In The Genes

There is a mountain of compelling science that supports the benefits of vegetables, and thanks to researchers from the British Institute of Food Research, we now know the science behind vegetables' "magical" effects. Reporting in the *Public Library of Science*, scientists found that vegetables' phytochemicals can directly incite hundreds of beneficial genetic changes. In the study, researchers had one group of men with pre-cancerous prostate lesions eat four extra servings of broccoli a week while a second group ate four extra servings of peas a week. Over the course of the one-year investigation, prostate tissue samples were monitored from both groups. Those that ate the broccoli had between 400 to 500 positive changes in genes known to fight cancer!

Broccoli and its cruciferous cousins (brussels sprouts, cabbage, kale, cauliflower, arugula and watercress) are uniquely high in two classes of phytochemicals, isothiocyanates and indoles. These phytochemicals have repeatedly displayed a championship anti-cancer performance in the lab. I urge everyone, especially those at high risk for cancer, to include a serving of cruciferous veggies in their diets every day.

This study also provides powerful confirmation that genes do not play the only role in disease formation. Genes are in constant interaction with the environment. In other words, your lifestyle (maintaining a healthy weight, eating right and being physically active) can have a tremendous impact—keeping good genes turned on and bad genes turned off.

Vision And Cognitive Decay

Our brains and eyes love fruits and veggies too, especially dark leafy greens. In a six-year study involving 3,700 elderly subjects, those who consumed two or more servings of vegetables a day had up to a 40 percent slower rate of cognitive decline. Those who consumed the most dark leafy greens fared the best in maintaining mental agility. For vision protection, leafy greens and citrus fruits are the consistent standouts. In a study evaluating the overall dietary pattern of 4,000 older adults in relation to age-related macular degeneration (a leading cause of adult blindness), those consuming the most dark leafy greens and citrus fruits had the lowest risk. A second study found men and women who ate three or more servings of fruit a day had a 36 percent lower risk of getting macular degeneration.

Canned Pumpkin Is **Great For You!**

Believe it or not, this convenient and inexpensive "canned" food is one of the healthiest ones available to you. It is fresh, pureed pumpkin, cooked down to remove its water, which concentrates its awesome nutritional attributes. Low in calories, high in fiber and providing the most potent package of disease-defying carotenoids known, canned pumpkin is an under-utilized superstar food. Add it to your soups, muffins, cornbread, and other baked goods. Put 2-3 tbs. in your morning oatmeal or yogurt and top it off with a dash or two of cinnamon for a sweeter kick.

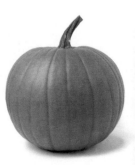

Spice up **your life!**

Get into the simple, tasty and super-healthy habit of adding herbs and spices to your foods. They add flavorful intrigue to almost any dish, (which means we can cut back on added fats, sauces and salt) and are virtually exploding with a seemingly endless list of beneficial phytochemicals. Here are my favorites:

 Parsley—This refreshing herb provides vitamin A, potassium, calcium, vitamin C and can boast a higher concentration of flavonoids than any other food! Flavonoids are powerful antioxidants that provide cardiovascular and cancer protection. You can grow your own parsley or buy it prepackaged. Add it to your favorite salads and pastas or go green with your rice dishes by adding a generous portion of chopped, fresh parsley.

 Rosemary—This savory herb contains phytochemicals that can reduce the amount of cancer-causing compounds known as heterocyclic amines (HCAs) that form in cooked meats. In addition, rosemary can enhance insulin sensitivity, which translates to a healthier metabolism. I always add a dash of dried rosemary or a tablespoon of fresh rosemary to my ground venison before grilling my burgers.

 Cilantro—This super flavorful herb contains a natural antibiotic called dodecanol. One study found that dodecanol killed the bacteria Salmonella more effectively than a powerful prescription antibiotic. Try adding cilantro to salsa for an extra tasty and healthy punch.

 Oregano—This is the perfect herb for adding Mediterranean flavor to your favorite dishes. Oregano is loaded with antioxidant power (up to 40 times more than apples). Add it to your salad dressings, include as a rub mixed with extra virgin olive oil on your chicken, or mix it with smashed avocado and lemon for a tasty substitute for mayonnaise on your sandwiches.

 Garlic—This popular spice contains medicinal plant compounds called allyl sulfides, which have been proven to boost the immune system. This makes garlic the perfect spice for cold and flu season. To maximize the goodness in garlic, use it freshly chopped or minced and add it to your foods at the end of cooking.

 Cinnamon—This sweet spice has recently won enthusiastic acclaim for its ability to boost insulin sensitivity and improve cholesterol and glucose metabolism. These properties may be especially beneficial for people with type 2 diabetes, pre-diabetes, weight issues and metabolic syndrome. Simply sprinkle cinnamon on to foods like cereals, oatmeal, yogurt, toast, cooked apples, coffee, hot cocoa, etc. One-half teaspoon is a good dose—I always add this amount to my morning cereal.

 Ginger—Ginger is packed with potent anti-inflammatory properties. Because excess inflammation is now widely recognized as a major contributor to many chronic diseases, ginger is one of the best all-around spices for disease prevention. The phytochemicals in ginger are also valuable for boosting immunity and for reducing nausea. For optimal results, include ginger in your diet regularly. Chop or grate fresh ginger root into sauces, salad dressings or right on top of your salad, poultry or seafood dishes. Drink freshly brewed tea steeped along with a small piece of chopped ginger. Dried powdered ginger is even more potent than fresh and can be used in cooking or sprinkled directly on to foods.

 Curry and Turmeric—These Indian spices are filled with a yellow pigment called curcumin which is one of the most potent natural anti-inflammatory agents ever identified. Several exciting studies are touting curry and turmeric for cancer protection, Alzheimer's protection and arthritis pain relief. For a boost of color and health, sprinkle curry or turmeric over bean dishes, poultry, tofu or rice.

 Hot Pepper—Spices made from hot peppers, like chili pepper, wasabi and cayenne pepper, can boost our mood. These hot spices stimulate the pain receptors in the mouth, which in turn triggers the release of endorphins—a natural morphine-like chemical that makes us feel good.

Lastly, although fresh herbs offer the most flavors and a higher concentration of antioxidants, dried herbs are still powerful and beneficial.

(Continued on page 72)

Make Room For **Mushrooms**

Although they are not technically a fruit or vegetable, mushrooms are great for you, and I encourage you to include them regularly in your diet. Mushrooms are low in calories (20 calories per ½ cup) and high in key nutrients, including B vitamins, copper, potassium and selenium. Additionally, a little known fact is that mushrooms are packed with powerful antioxidant chemicals. According to Penn State food scientist, Jay Dubost, mushrooms commonly found on grocery store shelves, like white buttons, criminis and portabellas, provide more antioxidant power than many vegetables. As an added bonus, mushrooms are especially high in beneficial polysaccharides, which enhance immune function.

Cooked mushrooms maintain their antioxidant capacity and make an excellent substitute for meat due to their savory flavor and hearty texture. I throw mushrooms into most of my salads, soups, stews, spaghetti and pasta sauces as a quick and simple way to boost my meal's nutritional value.

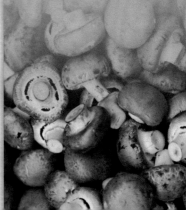

The more colorful the food, the more it's packed with valuable nutrients. Eat from the entire spectrum to fully leverage the tens of thousands of beneficial compounds these foods offer. Remember, color means health: the deeper and richer the color, the more phytochemicals, vitamins and minerals present in the food.

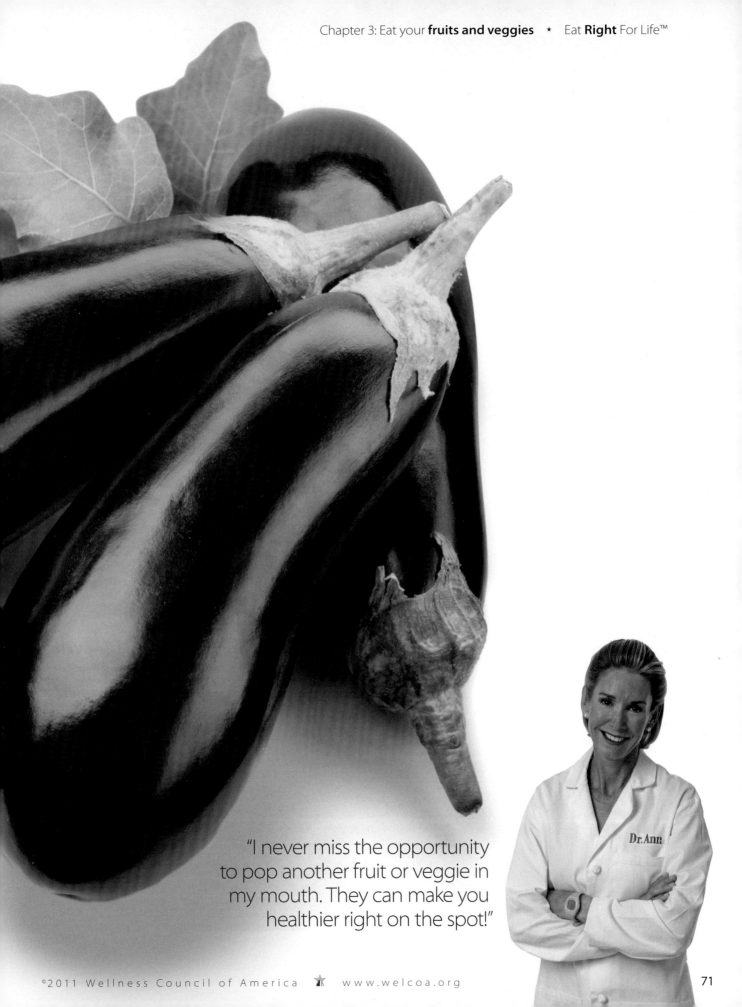

"I never miss the opportunity to pop another fruit or veggie in my mouth. They can make you healthier right on the spot!"

Eat More, Weigh Less

When it comes to fruits and veggies, you can really eat more to weigh less! The more of them you eat, the leaner you will be.

Fruits and non-starchy vegetables are naturally slimming foods because they contain large amounts of zero calorie water and fiber. This combination is critical for weight loss and maintenance, as volume trumps calories when it comes to satisfying the desire for food. Filling your stomach with a certain volume of food can shut off the brain's appetite center regardless of how many calories it has. In fact, it appears that our bodies desire a given volume of food over a certain number of calories. This reality is invaluable for controlling hunger and appetite. Therefore, for weight loss and maintenance, you should always look to add fruits and non-starchy veggies to your meals.

Let me give you a simple example to make this point: If you ate a plate piled with steamed broccoli, you would feel satisfied (likely even stuffed) from its volume, yet would have only consumed about 130 calories. Indeed, this is a highly effective strategy that has been proven in many scientific studies. One weight loss study found that the most successful participants reduced caloric density by consuming more fruits and vegetables. These participants shed more than twice as much weight as those who reduced their caloric density the least. What's more, the study group who lost the most weight actually ate more food—about 10½ ounces more daily. In a study evaluating the diets of 7,500 "typical" Americans, those who ate the most fruits and vegetables ate more food by weight, yet weighed less. Another study presented at the same meeting found that study subjects instructed to eat more fruits and vegetables lost more weight without counting calories and without feeling like they were dieting than the control group who was put on a strict diet that reduced portion sizes and fat intake.

Dr. Ann's Fundamental Theorem Of Flavor

To improve the health and the taste of your diet, it's important to constantly tell yourself how good healthy foods are and how harmful the unhealthy ones are for your body. If you do, the good will taste better and the bad will taste worse. Try it, it works!

Getting The Most Nutritional Bang For Your Buck
At The Salad Bar

Five Rules To Follow

Well-stocked salad bars offer a quick and convenient opportunity to tap into the nutritional excellence fruits and vegetables provide. To successfully navigate through the salad bar and get the most nutritional bang for your buck, keep the following five rules in mind.

BEGIN WITH A BASE OF HEALTHY GREENS.
- Go for those with the deepest green color. The more color, the more disease-busting phytochemicals, vitamins and minerals it will have. Baby spinach is my top pick followed by romaine and mixed mescaline greens.
- Keep in mind that iceberg lettuce offers minimal nutritional value.

ADD AS MANY RICHLY COLORED FRUITS AND VEGGIES AS POSSIBLE.
- Salad bar superstars include red onions, carrots, broccoli florets, tomatoes, bell peppers, olives, berries, cantaloupe and red grapes.
- Remember, fruits and vegetables are the best option for those who want high nutrient content and satiety with low calories.

ALWAYS INCLUDE APPROXIMATELY 3 OUNCES OF HEALTHY, LEAN PROTEIN FOR LONGER LASTING APPETITE CONTROL.
- Three ounces is about the size of your palm. Your best choices include skinless turkey or chicken, hard-cooked eggs or low-fat cottage cheese. Shrimp and fish are also fantastic, if available.
- Vegetable-protein alternatives are an excellent choice and include tofu squares, chick peas or other beans, and nuts and seeds (almonds, walnuts, sunflower seeds, pumpkin seeds, pine nuts, etc.).

TOP YOUR SALAD WITH THE DRESSING KNOWN TO PROTECT YOUR HEALTH AND YOUR HEART—OLIVE OIL AND VINEGAR.
- If not available, choose a reduced-fat variety or vinaigrette.
- Avoid the thicker, creamier varieties—they are generally made from a less-healthy oil base—and stay away from fat-free as they are high in sugar.

AVOID THE "WHITE STUFF"—PASTA SALADS, POTATO SALADS, CROUTONS, CHICKEN SALADS, ETC.
- We covered the "Great White Hazards" in the previous chapter, so you know these foods are not good for you!

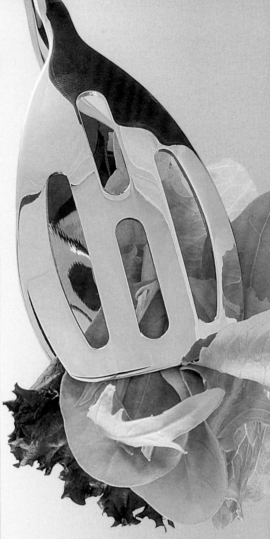

Go Green!
Dark leafy greens are Mother Nature's multivitamin. Be sure to include some form of them in your diet each day. You can choose from collards, kale, spinach, and a wide variety of lettuce greens.

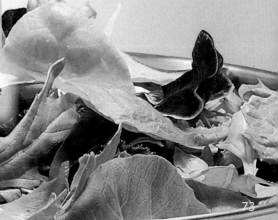

Salad bars are fantastic when you make the right choices. Take heed of these five rules and your next trip to the salad buffet will be a healthful one.

When it comes to fruits and veggies, you really can eat more and weigh less. So, load your meals and snacks up with as much high fiber, high water fruits and veggies as possible. In this regard, your very best choices include the following:

Fruits: berries, cherries, plums, any whole citrus, melon, grapes, peaches, apples, pears and kiwi (avoid "low volume" dried fruits)

Vegetables: cabbage, kale, broccoli, cauliflower, brussels sprouts, collards, carrots, garlic, onions, leeks, tomatoes, asparagus, spinach, dark lettuces, bell peppers and mushrooms

Here are some easy tips and strategies for success:

- Double up your fruit and vegetable side dishes

- Feature veggies as your main dish

- Fill the majority of your plate up with veggies before serving the rest of your meal

- Substitute a non-starchy vegetable for the side of potatoes

- If veggies are called for in recipes, throw in extra

- Slice up fresh fruits and vegetables at night and snack on them the next day

If you're weight-conscious, fruits and vegetables are a supreme choice. Not only do they satisfy the appetite, but they are also low in calories. Load up!

Always Focus On Fruits And Vegetables

When buying, ordering or preparing your food always think of fruits and vegetables! Make them your focus. For best results, strive for seven or more servings of fruits and veggies (total) a day. A serving is one-half cup in any form with the exception of raw, leafy greens. A serving of leafy greens is one cup uncooked. Because vegetables have a slight edge over fruit in terms of nutrient density and providing a lower glycemic response (fruits have some natural sugars), it's best to include them more often. If you need to lose weight or have diabetes, pre-diabetes or metabolic syndrome, be especially vigilant in eating as many non-starchy vegetables as you can and limit fruit to less than three servings a day.

Although seven servings is the ultimate daily goal, please don't view this as an all-or-nothing recommendation. Fruits and vegetables are so potent that any improvement you can make—even adding just a single serving a day—is valuable to your health.

Use the following *Eat Your Fruits And Veggies Plan Of Action* to help you in your healthy quest to include as many and as much variety of these remarkable foods as possible.

PLAN OF ACTION Eat your **fruits and veggies**.

1. VEGETABLES

- **Consume five or more servings a day.** The more the better, but any improvement is great.
  - ➤ A serving is one-half cup of any vegetable, except dark leafy greens.
  - ➤ For dark leafy greens, (spinach, lettuce, collards, etc.) one serving is one cup uncooked.
  - ➤ Dark, leafy greens are the most nutrient dense, disease-protective foods nature offers. Be sure to include them in your daily diet. Eat a big green salad with a variety of veggies at least once a day.

- **Focus on the superstars**—All cruciferous veggies (cabbage, kale, broccoli, cauliflower, brussels sprouts and collards), carrots, garlic, onions, leeks, tomatoes, asparagus, sweet potatoes, dark leafy salad greens (like spinach), and red, orange and yellow bell peppers.

- **Eat your vegetables fresh or frozen**, but try to avoid frozen veggies with added butter or sauces as well as canned vegetables, as they have inferior nutritional quality and excess sodium. Canned pumpkin, tomatoes, tomato products, roasted red peppers, olives, beans and artichokes are an exception, so include them freely.

- **Minimize the starchy, higher glycemic vegetables:** potatoes, parsnips, rutabagas and corn (avoid this group if overweight, diabetic, pre-diabetic or if you have metabolic syndrome).

- **Use fresh and/or dried herbs and spices in your food preparation.** They kick up the flavor of your food for zero calories and are exploding with health-boosting phytochemicals.

- **Snack on fresh veggies** (carrots, celery, bell peppers and broccoli florets). Dip in a healthy dip like hummus, salsa or guacamole.

- **Cook veggies by steaming, pan-sautéing or roasting.** Avoid boiling.

2. FRUIT

- **Strive for two or more servings of fruit a day.**
  - ➤ A serving is one-half cup fresh or frozen or ¼ cup dried.
  - ➤ If diabetic or overweight, include fruit daily, but limit to two servings. Avoid dried fruit (the exception is apricots) and the sweeter, high glycemic tropical fruits (bananas, pineapple, mangos and papayas).

- **Concentrate on the superstars**—berries (any variety), cherries, plums, any whole citrus, cantaloupe, red/purple grapes, peaches, apples, pears, kiwi, dried or fresh apricots.

- **Enjoy fresh or frozen as long as they contain no added sugar.**

- **Avoid canned fruits**, as they are nutritionally inferior and often have added sugar.

- **Snack on fresh fruit.**

- **Choose fresh fruit for dessert.**

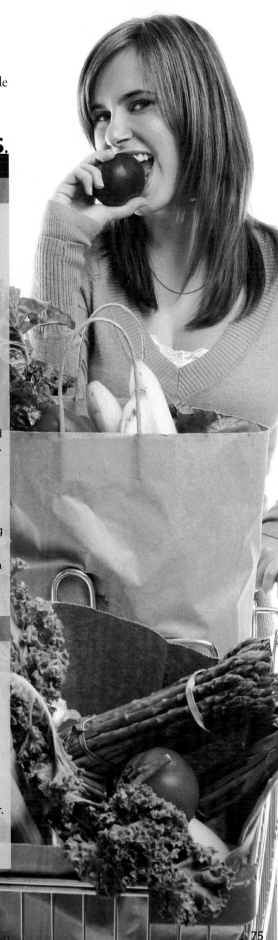

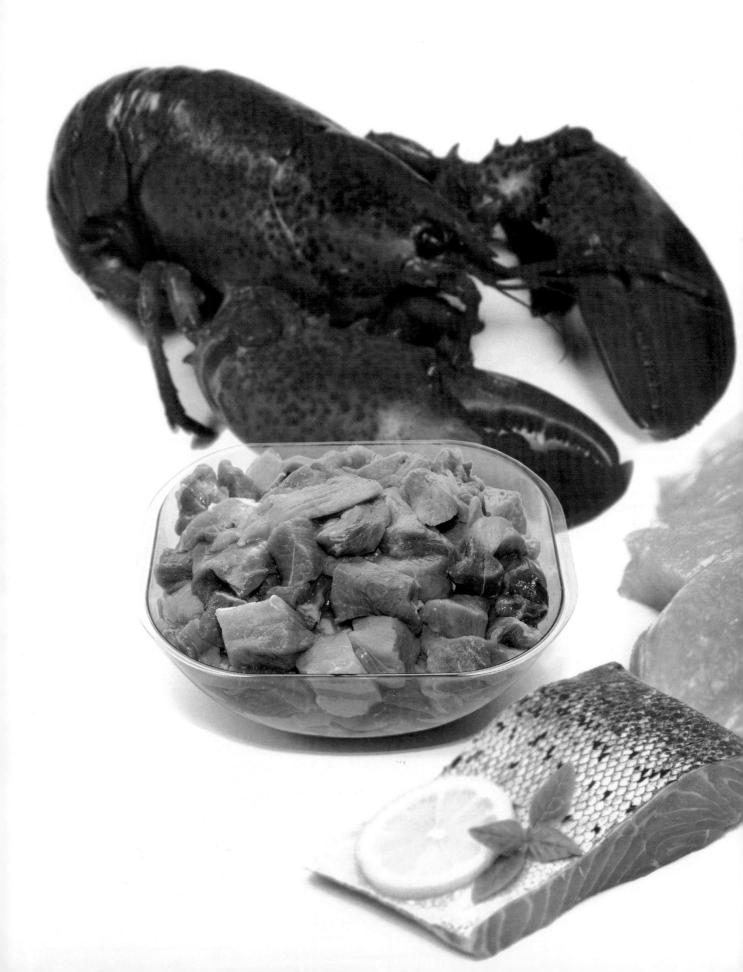

[CHAPTER 4]
Select the **right** proteins

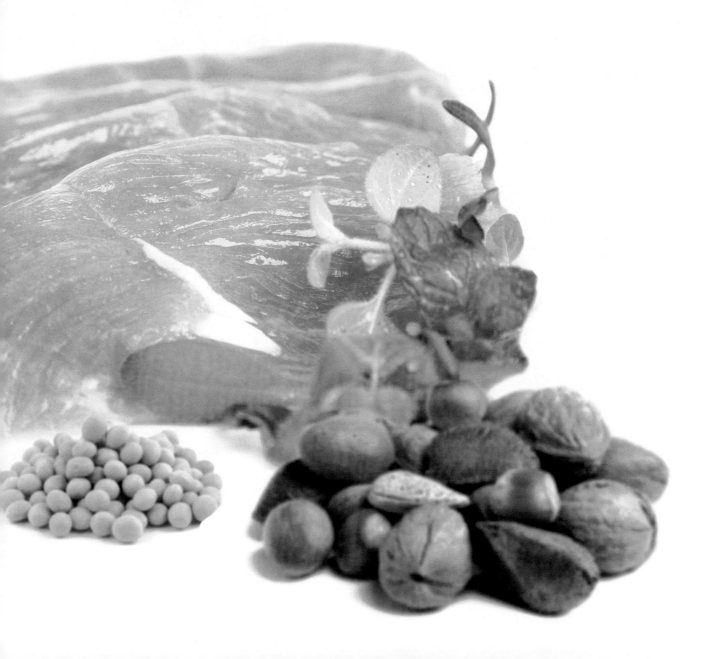

[CHAPTER 4]

Select the **right** proteins

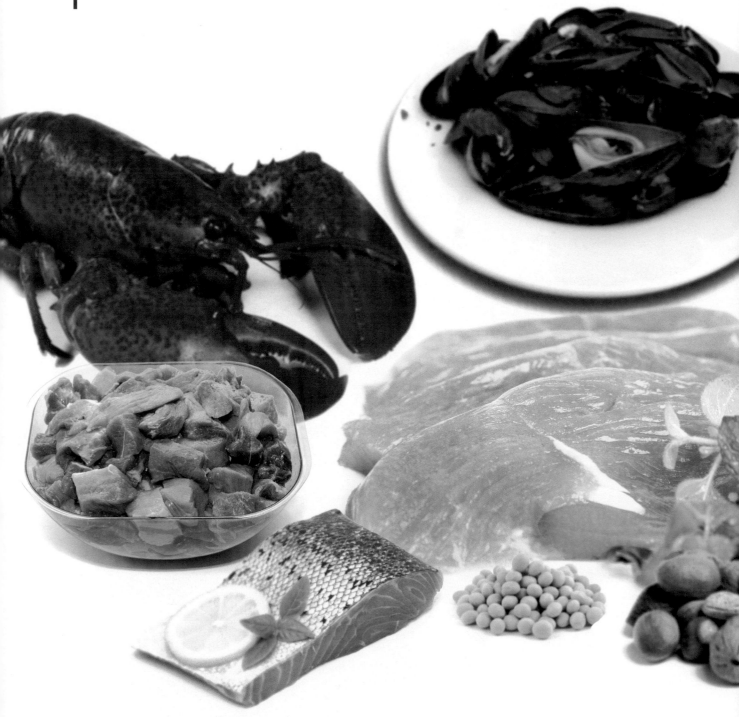

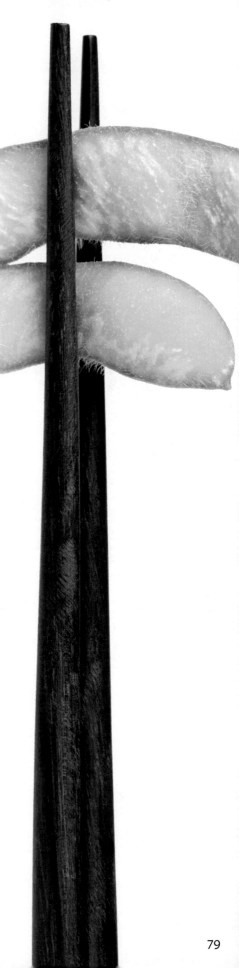

The right proteins are a powerful ally in your pursuit of optimal wellness and vitality. When it comes to dietary protein and eating right for life, there are two primary rules you need to follow. First, you need to select the right form of protein. Second, you should always include some form of healthy protein at each meal.

Just like fats and carbs, some proteins are better for you than others. The healthiest proteins contain health-promoting nutrients like omega-3 fats and phytochemicals, and are largely free of components like trans fats and saturated fats. Let's look at a few basic examples for clarification.

How A Healthy Protein Breaks Down

A six-ounce broiled Porterhouse steak is a great source of protein—38 grams worth. But it also delivers 44 grams of fat, 16 of which are saturated—that's almost three-fourths of the FDA recommended daily intake for saturated fat! Now let's take a look at a healthy protein. The same portion of salmon provides 34 grams of protein, four grams of saturated fat and 18 grams of good fat. Another healthy protein includes lentils. A cup of cooked lentils has 34 grams of protein, delivers less than one gram of fat and is loaded with fiber, vitamins, minerals and disease-fighting phytochemicals.

Indeed, nature has graciously provided a long list of delicious, healthy proteins from which to choose. They include the following:

- Fish, especially the oily varieties
- Shellfish
- Poultry
- Eggs, especially omega-3 fortified
- Nuts and seeds
- Beans
- Wild game
- Low-fat dairy products
- Whole soy foods

You don't have to commit this list of healthy proteins to memory. Just know that there are two much-less-healthy proteins, and if you restrict these two proteins, any other proteins you eat should be fine. The two proteins you should limit are:

1. Red meat, especially fatty cuts and processed varieties

2. Full-fat dairy products

We will switch things up a bit in this section, and discuss the healthy proteins first.

My Favorite "Convenience" Food

One of my favorite convenience foods is single-serving pouches of shelf-stable wild Alaskan salmon. You can find it at most grocers in the canned seafood section. I top my lunch salad at least twice a week with this superstar protein. Each three-ounce serving provides 1,000 milligrams of omega-3 fats, 13 grams of protein and over 100 percent of the recommended daily amount of vitamin D—all for just 120 calories!

THE HEALTHY PROTEINS
Fish: A Good Catch

The data is simply overwhelming that fish is good for us. Populations that eat more fish have fewer cases of heart disease, cancer, depression, arthritis, impotence and Alzheimer's. Fish, especially the oily varieties like salmon and sardines, are one of the healthiest proteins on earth. They provide complete protein (all of the essential amino acids) along with several key nutrients, including magnesium, selenium, potassium, vitamin D and B vitamins. Fish also deliver heart-healthy omega-3 fats.

The Double Duty Benefits Of Fish

Studies have shown that eating fish is one of the most powerful things you can do to guard your heart and brain. A fascinating report in the *Journal of the American College of Cardiology* found that the fish in traditional Japanese diets is likely the secret weapon for their "puzzlingly low" rates of heart disease. Investigators measured the amount of calcium (a marker for heart disease) in the coronary arteries of 869 Japanese and U.S. middle-aged men. Although the Japanese men had much higher rates of smoking and equivalent rates of other cardiovascular risk factors, like high blood pressure and diabetes, they had much lower rates (about three times less) of calcium build-up in their arteries compared to the U.S. males. The one distinctive difference between the two groups: the Japanese men had twice the amount of omega-3 fats in their blood. Of course, these findings aren't too surprising since we know that omega-3 fats provide seven separate cardiovascular benefits. In another study that included more than 43,000 adult males, those who reported eating fish as little as one to three times a month were 43 percent less likely to suffer an ischemic stroke (the most common type of stroke) versus those who never ate fish.

And fish really is brain food. A report in the journal *Neurology* found that older adults who regularly included fish in their diets had healthier brain structure. In this study, 3,660 elderly subjects were followed over a five-year period. Those who ate baked or broiled fish at least three times a week were 25 percent less likely to have areas of subtle brain damage (brain infarcts). Brain infarcts are powerful predictors of strokes and dementia.

The omega-3 fats in fish help ensure that your brain gets the steady and robust blood flow it requires by keeping arteries healthy and well-functioning. Omega-3s in fish also provide the brain with the fatty acid, DHA. DHA, better known as the smart fat, has been shown to effectively ward off

Alzheimer's and other forms of dementia. A study that included more than 15,000 elderly subjects from seven different countries found that those who enjoyed fish most or all days of the week were 38 percent less likely to develop dementia versus those who rarely ate fish.

Go Fish!

Fish is ultimately one of the most nutritious, highest quality sources of protein available, and I encourage you to make it a regular part of your diet. You should strive for at least two servings of fish in your diet each week. The oily varieties offer a hearty supply of long-chained omega-3 fats, DHA and EPA, and are your best options. Breaded, deep-fried fish and fish sticks do not count, so stick to baked, broiled, poached and pan-seared.

Other Proteins In The Sea: Shellfish

Shrimp, clams, oysters, scallops and lobster offer a delectable and super-healthy alternative to red meat and are low in calories and bad fats. Shellfish are brimming with nourishment including B vitamins, vitamin D, and those awesome omega-3 fats. They are rich in an array of important minerals and provide more zinc than any other food. Contrary to popular belief, shellfish do not have adverse effects on overall cholesterol levels and have been shown to actually benefit cardiovascular health, especially when eaten in lieu of fatty red meats.

Poultry: Protein With A Punch

In a striking contrast to red meat, chicken and turkey have never been directly associated with chronic diseases and provide an abundance of nutritional goodness. When you get your protein from poultry, you also get a nice dose of several B vitamins, iron, selenium and zinc. Further, as opposed to red meats, the flesh of poultry comes largely devoid of artery-clogging saturated fats. Three ounces of skinless turkey or chicken breast provide 26 grams of protein and less than one gram of saturated fat; while three ounces of standard ground beef provide 20 grams of protein and four and a half grams of saturated fat. For best results, choose baked, broiled or roasted chicken and turkey. If weight is an issue, remove the skin before you eat it. And just say no to the fried versions!

Avoid The "Dirty" Fish

Certain types of fish are high in environmental toxins like polychlorinated biphenyls (PCBs), dioxins and methyl mercury, and should be avoided. These include the larger, longer-living carnivorous species, such as shark, marlin, king mackerel, tile fish and sword fish. Fresh tuna and canned white Albacore tuna can be moderately high in methyl mercury. I recommend you limit these forms of tuna to two servings per month. School-age children as well as women who are pregnant, nursing or may become pregnant are uniquely vulnerable to these toxins and should avoid fresh and canned white Albacore tuna altogether. Canned chunk lite tuna has less mercury and is acceptable in moderation.

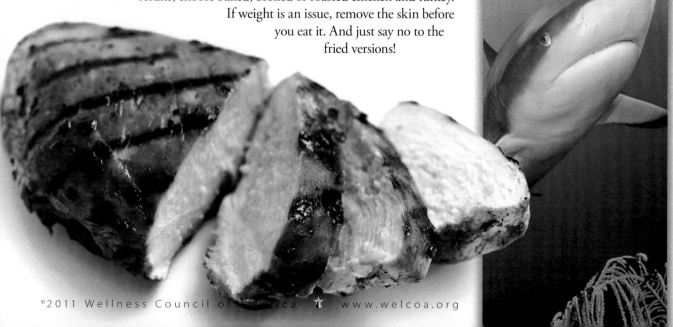

Shrimp, clams, oysters, scallops and lobster offer a delectable and super-healthy alternative to red meat and are low in calories and bad fats. Shellfish are brimming with nourishment including B vitamins, vitamin D, and those awesome omega-3 fats.

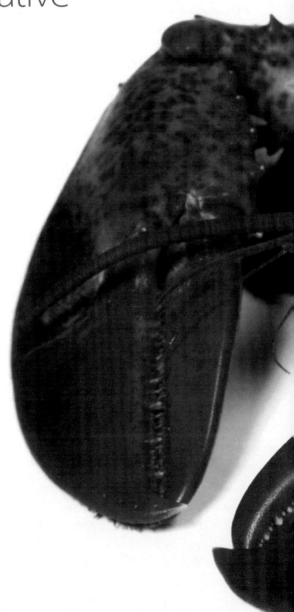

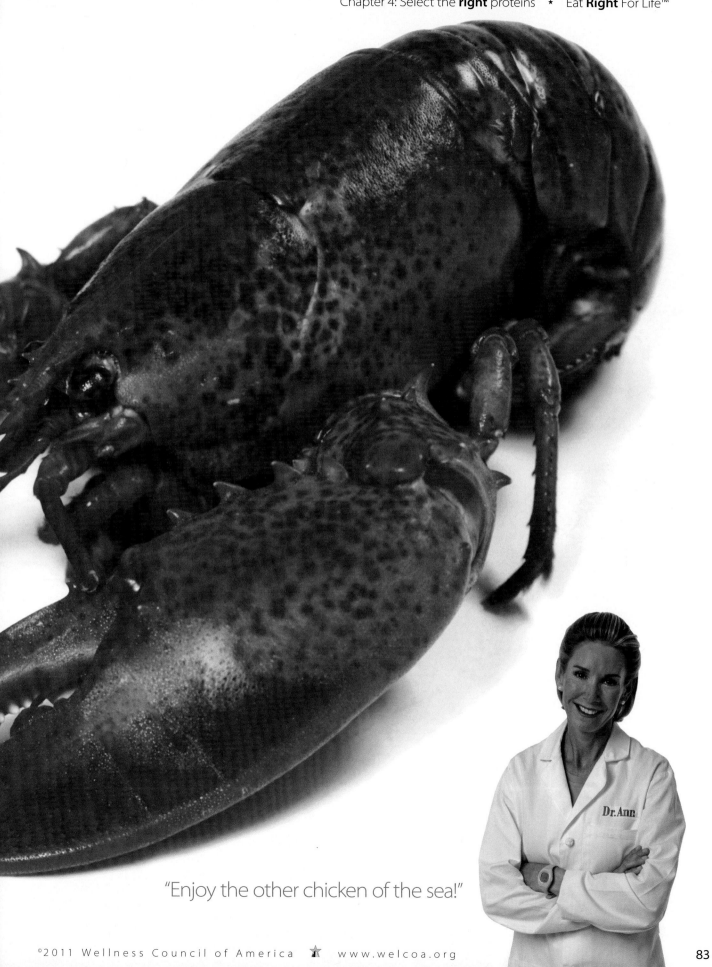

"Enjoy the other chicken of the sea!"

Soy Nuts: Good And
Good For You

If you are one of the 74 million Americans who have high blood pressure, soy nuts may be a particularly good snack selection. A fascinating clinical trial found that a half-cup of roasted soy nuts consumed over the course of the day lowered blood pressure to the same degree as standard blood pressure medications. Eating soy nuts was also effective in reducing the blood pressure of people with pre-hypertension, defined as blood pressure between 120/80—139/89. Maintaining normal blood pressure—ideally 115/75 or less—is paramount to staying healthy. Even the lowest levels of pre-hypertension (120/80) can increase the risk of cardiovascular disease two and a half fold!

Roasted soy nuts are delicious, inexpensive and highly nutritious. You can find them in most standard grocers—try them!

Soy: Scoop it Up

There is perhaps no other group of foods that have received more spin than soy, and it seems to have generated a lot of confusion. Whole soy foods fit beautifully into the mix of healthy proteins. Here are the soy food facts based on the latest science:

1. Whole soy foods have an exemplary nutritional profile—they are very nutritious foods.
   - Soy foods provide high quality complete vegetable-based protein that is naturally low in saturated fat and cholesterol-free.
   - Soy foods are rich in essential nutrients including B vitamins, vitamin E, calcium, magnesium, iron, potassium and selenium.
   - Soy foods are high in soluble fiber—the fiber that reduces cholesterol and stabilizes blood sugar.
   - Soy foods provide heart-healthy fats, including the superstar omega-3 fats.
   - Soy foods provide an abundance of disease-fighting phytochemicals including isoflavones, saponins, phytosterols and protease inhibitors.

2. When consumed regularly (especially when they replace foods high in saturated fats like red meat) whole soy foods have been shown to modestly lower LDL (bad) cholesterol levels.

3. Regular consumption of soy foods has been associated with lower rates of cancer including breast, colon, prostate, lung and endometrial cancer. Regular consumption of whole soy foods has been associated with protection from osteoporosis and a reduction in fracture risk.

4. Regular consumption of soy foods may diminish menopausal symptoms in women.

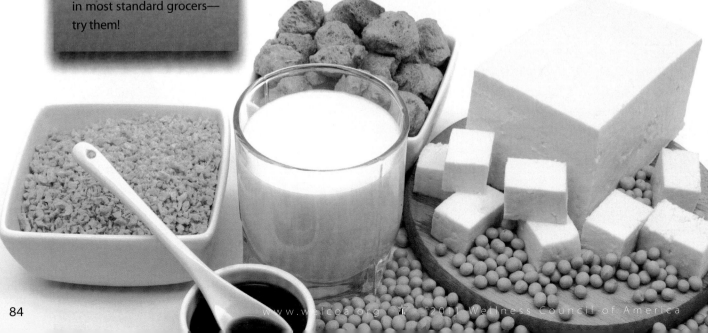

Bottom line: everyone can benefit from the stellar package of nutrients whole soy foods provide. Whole soy foods include edamame, tofu, tempeh, soy milk, miso, roasted soy nuts and soy flour. I recommend you include the ones you like as part of your well-balanced diet. In my experience, most everyone (including kids) find edamame (fresh green soybeans) and roasted soy nuts delicious. Tempeh and tofu are bland and tasteless on their own, but can readily adapt to the flavor of whatever you add to them—teriyaki, barbecue, vinegar, etc. My personal favorite is tempeh—a fermented form of soy that has a firm, cheese-like texture. I flavor it with a little extra virgin olive oil, balsamic vinegar, salt and pepper and add it to salads and wraps. Regardless of the soy foods you choose, I recommend organic, non-GMO varieties. Additionally, you should avoid soy supplements and soy pills, as their safety has not been established.

Eggs: Break Them Out Of Their Shells

Eggs have always been a delicious and convenient source of high-quality, low-fat protein and, thanks to modern food technology, eggs are healthier than ever these days. Along with B vitamins, vitamin E, and iron, you can even get omega-3 fats in your eggs. Many egg producers are fortifying their chicken feed with omega-3 fats, which means that this superstar fat gets incorporated into the egg yolk. These omega-3 eggs are available at most grocery stores. You will pay a bit more, but it's well worth it, as these eggs are second only to seafood as the most plentiful food source of DHA. Simply look for "DHA" or "omega-3" on the label. Eggland's Best is a popular national brand that has also been voted America's "best-tasting" egg by the American Culinary Institute.

Eggs are healthiest if prepared boiled or poached. I always keep a carton of boiled eggs at home in my refrigerator for a great, grab-and-go protein source.

Wild Game: Hunt These Proteins Down

If you have access to it, wild game definitely has its rightful place in a healthy diet. After all, our hunter-gatherer ancestors who by most accounts did not develop chronic diseases consumed it regularly. Deer, antelope, moose, duck, goose, pheasant, turkey, quail and dove are excellent sources of high-quality, lean protein. Due to their natural diets and wild habitats, the nutritional profiles of wild game are very different from their domesticated counterparts. Wild game has fewer calories, less total fat and less saturated fat than their factory-farmed versions. Wild animals are free of potentially harmful added ingredients, like antibiotics and hormones, and they are plentiful in beneficial fats, including omega-3s. For perspective, consider that a wild cape buffalo living and eating in its natural environment provides one-tenth the total fat, half the saturated fat and up to six times more omega-3 fats than a grain-fed, domesticated modern day steer.

All About Eggs And Cholesterol

Please know that there is no scientific evidence that eggs elevate the risk of cardiovascular disease in healthy subjects. However, there is some evidence that eggs can elevate cholesterol levels and increase cardiovascular risk in people who already have high cholesterol levels and/or are diabetic. I recommend that diabetics and those with cardiovascular risk factors limit eggs to less than five a week.

See The Benefits Of Eggs

One of eggs' most important yet barely recognized health benefits relates to preservation of eyesight. Egg yolks provide the most bio-available form of lutein. Lutein is a carotenoid phytochemical that shields the eyes from the damaging effects of sunlight. Eggs provide about three times higher blood levels of lutein than most other food sources, which ultimately protects the eyes from age-related macular degeneration and cataracts.

High On Hemp

I am frequently asked what protein powder I recommend, and finally I have discovered one that I know is truly "healthy" and that I can wholeheartedly endorse—hemp seed powder. It is made from ground hemp seeds so it is a "whole food" protein versus the "isolated" protein in whey, casein, or soy-based protein powders. Hemp seeds provide high quality "complete" protein that is gentler on your bones, your digestive system, and the environment. Additionally, hemp seeds are one of the most nutritionally complete foods on the planet. Aside from a whopping dose of protein and fiber, ground hemp seeds provide all the essential fatty acids, including a big hit of omega-3 along with B vitamins, vitamins D and E, and a comprehensive package of minerals. The "all natural" nutritional firepower in hemp seed powder puts the others to shame. Unlike marijuana leaves—hemp seeds do not contain any THC. You can find it in healthy grocery stores. Be sure to select 100% ground hemp seeds vs hemp protein powder—you want the full package of nutritional excellence the seeds provide.

Protein Is Nature's Diet Pill

Of the three basic building blocks of nutrition—protein, carbohydrates and fat—nothing provides longer-lasting and more effective appetite control than protein. In fact, I like to call protein nature's diet pill!

There are many reasons why protein helps stave off hunger. When proteins are digested, they produce a prolonged and steady level of glucose in the bloodstream. This keeps your brain's appetite center in the "off" position longer than if you were to eat a carbohydrate or fat-laden meal. Foods that are rich in protein also slow the overall digestive process by delaying gastric emptying. This means that foods will stay in your stomach longer, enhancing the feeling of fullness and satiety. Lastly, protein is more effective than carbs and fats when it comes to deceasing levels of the powerful hunger-generating hormone, ghrelin. Ghrelin is produced by cells that line your stomach and it's your body's appetite-stimulating hormone. The lower your ghrelin level, the less hungry you will feel.

Take full advantage of protein's appetite-suppressive effects by getting enough of it at each meal. Here are some tips that will help you in that effort:

- Include a nice dose (12 grams or more) of protein at each meal.
  - ➤ The right dose should give you at least two hours of satiety (appetite suppression).
  - ➤ If you are hungry less than two hours after a meal, you need to increase your protein a bit.
  - ➤ The best protein choices for your health and your waistline include fish, shellfish, skinless poultry, nuts, seeds, whole soy foods, low-fat or skim dairy products, omega-3 eggs, and beans and legumes.

- Make sure you get adequate protein at breakfast.
  - ➤ Getting adequate protein at breakfast appears to be particularly valuable for appetite control.
  - ➤ To get the healthiest, leanest sources of protein at breakfast, try a veggie omelet topped with skim or reduced fat cheese; a fruit smoothie with a couple of scoops of ground hemp seeds; a whole wheat bagel topped with some peanut butter or smoked salmon; a bowl of high protein cereal and skim or soy milk topped with a handful of nuts; some low-fat cottage cheese with fresh fruit; or a whole grain breakfast burrito with eggs, beans and salsa.

No doubt about it—eating the right proteins can help us feel energized and full, all without the extra calories and fat. So ditch the diet pills and get the real!

Can You Get Too Much Protein?

Too little protein is clearly a problem, but what about too much? Protein is an essential nutrient required for cell maintenance and repair as well as the regulation of bodily functions. The amount of protein we need largely depends on our age, lean body mass, activity level and health status. The average adult female requires about 50 grams a day, and the average adult male needs about 65 grams a day. However, the average American female consumes about 70 grams a day, while the average male gets about 100 grams a day. A cup of yogurt at breakfast (12 grams), three ounces of tuna at lunch (20 grams), four ounces of chicken at dinner (28 grams), and a one-ounce snack of almonds (6 grams) would suffice.

Consuming excessive amounts of protein, as recommended by some low-carb diet plans, should be avoided, especially over the long term. As a normal by-product of protein metabolism, acid is released into the bloodstream after protein is consumed. This acid has to be neutralized or buffered, and the body uses calcium for this purpose. If there is not sufficient calcium in the bloodstream, it is taken directly from bones to perform this task. The kidneys then excrete these calcium-acid waste products through the urine. It is well established that high-protein diets promote urinary excretion of calcium. A short-term commitment to a high-protein diet is unlikely to have a significant effect on bone health, but adhering to this type of diet for an extended period of time may very well compromise bone integrity and can predispose a person to osteoporosis. In the Nurses' Health Study, women who ate more than 95 grams of protein a day were 20 percent more likely to have broken a wrist over a 12-year period compared to those who ate an average amount of protein (less than 68 grams a day).

As already mentioned, the kidneys are responsible for releasing the acidic by-products of protein metabolism. When faced with excessive protein loads, the kidneys indeed may be overtaxed. A Harvard-based study found that high-protein diets in women, particularly from meat, increased the rate of kidney decline in those with pre-existing mild kidney dysfunction. The elderly and those with high blood pressure, diabetes, gout and obesity are at high risk for mild kidney dysfunction and should avoid long-term use of high-protein diet plans.

Protein Put To The Test

To test the power of protein, researchers at the University of Washington School of Medicine placed 19 study subjects on different diets, each with a varying protein content. In the first phase, the study subjects were placed on a two-week weight-maintenance diet. On that diet, 15 percent of their calories came from protein, 35 percent came from fat, and 50 percent came from carbohydrates. In phase two, they were transitioned to a two-week diet consisting of the same number of calories, but with more protein and less fat (30 percent from protein, 20 percent from fat and 50 percent from carbohydrates). Then the study subjects spent the final 12-week phase eating whatever they wanted, while maintaining the same percentages of calories from foods (again, 30 percent from protein, 20 percent from fat and 50 percent from carbs).

The results? Study subjects reported a markedly decreased appetite while on the higher protein phase two diet. During phase three, despite the fact that they could eat whatever they wanted, study subjects ate 450 less calories and lost 11 pounds on average.

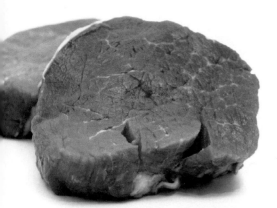

THE NOT SO HEALTHY PROTEINS
Red Meat

I actually love red meat, but because it has such a bad rap, I include it in my diet sparingly. Red meat, which includes beef, pork and lamb can include a host of harmful substances, including excessive amounts of heme-iron, carcinogens, arachidonic acid, oxycholesterol, excess omega-6 fats, antibiotic residues, environmental toxins (pesticides, PCBs, dioxins) and hormone residues like IGF-1.

My Beef With Red Meat

I include red meat in my diet, but I make a concerted effort to limit it to two servings or less a week. Here are seven great reasons to follow my lead and curtail your intake of red meat.

(1) **Red meat contains lots of saturated fat.** Eating excessive saturated fat can increase your risk of heart disease and promote insulin resistance.

(2) **Red meat is a rich food source of arachidonic acid.** Arachidonic acid is an infamous, pro-inflammatory fatty acid. As I've mentioned, inflammation plays a prominent role in the development of cardiovascular disease, Alzheimer's disease, allergies, asthma, autoimmune conditions and some forms of cancer. Additionally, a landmark study published in the *New England Journal of Medicine* found that six percent of Americans carry a gene variant that dramatically increases their risk of heart disease, especially when foods high in arachidonic acid (red meat) are consumed.

(3) **Red meat from domesticated animals contains lots of omega-6 fatty acids and minimal to no omega-3 fatty acids.** Omega-6 fatty acids compete in the body with omega-3 fatty acids. All domesticated livestock, with the exception of those that are free range, are fed artificial diets heavy in omega-6 fats. Excessive consumption of red meat contributes to an unhealthy omega-6, omega-3 fatty acid ratio.

(4) **Heavy red meat consumption has been associated with several forms of cancer.** A potent class of known carcinogens (cancer-causing agents) called heterocyclic amines form within the protein fibers of red meat when heated at high temperatures (grilling, barbecuing and frying). A second class of carcinogens, nitrosamines, can form in the gastrointestinal tract from sodium nitrite contained in processed and cured meats (bacon, ham, salami, bologna, hot dogs, and other processed luncheon meats).

(5) **Red meat (especially beef) contains high concentrations of iron.** Iron from red meat, unlike vegetable sources of iron, is absorbed from the gastrointestinal tract whether the body needs it or not. Excessive iron in the bloodstream behaves as a potent pro-oxidant and has been implicated in promoting heart disease, breast cancer, colon cancer and type 2 diabetes.

(6) **Red meat contains potentially harmful added ingredients.** Virtually all domesticated livestock (with the exception of those deemed organic or free range) contain antibiotic and sex steroid hormonal residues. Excessive exposure to these chemicals may predispose humans to resistant bacterial pathogens as well as hormonally sensitive cancers, like breast, prostate and ovarian Moreover, eating red meat increases your exposure to harmful agents such as pesticides, herbicides, heavy metals, PCBs and dioxins.

(7) **Red meat may contain harmful viruses and bacteria.** Undercooked red meat can lead to potentially life-threatening infections.

The scientific research linking diets heavy in red meat and increased disease risk is rich and voluminous. Having reviewed thousands of diet and nutrition studies over the past decade, I cannot recall a single one that reported any disease protection from eating red meat. On the contrary, my files are filled with reports that show a consistent and clear relationship between consuming red meat and a multitude of health problems, including heart disease, stroke, type 2 diabetes, obesity, and many forms of cancer. Here is a snapshot of some of the most compelling studies to date:

- The largest study ever conducted to establish the health effects of eating red meat found that those consuming the most red meat—about a quarter-pound hamburger or a pork chop a day—were more likely to develop a number of different cancers, including colorectal, esophageal, liver, lung, pancreatic and advanced prostate cancer. This eight-year evaluation included over 500,000 adults from 10 different European countries.

- In a study involving 284 middle-aged women, those who consumed the most red meat were more likely to be obese. Of those consuming three or more servings a day, about 53 percent were obese. Of those consuming less than two servings a day, only 15 percent were obese.

- After following the diets of over half a million adults over the course of 10 years, men and women consuming the most red meat had a 31 and 36 percent, respectively, higher risk of dying from all causes compared to those consuming the least. In this evaluation, the risk of cardiovascular disease was 27 percent higher for men and 50 percent higher for women eating the most red meat.

- Processed red meat appears to be particularly risky, especially for colon cancer. A large review of 24 studies found that for every one-ounce increase of processed red meat (bacon, sausage, ham, etc.) consumed daily, the risk of colon cancer increased by almost 49 percent.

- In a prospective study involving over 37,000 women followed for more than eight years, those who ate the most red meat were 28 percent more likely to develop type 2 diabetes than study subjects who consumed the least. In this evaluation, bacon and hot dogs were the most risky of all types of red meat.

I recommend that you limit red meat, which includes beef, pork and lamb, to two servings or less a week. When you have it, go for the leanest cuts, like tenderloin and sirloin. Be especially vigilant in restricting processed varieties like bacon, bologna and sausage.

(Continued on page 92)

Beware Of Oxycholesterol

Scientists from the Chinese University of Hong Kong have uncovered perhaps the most compelling reason to eliminate fried foods from your diet: oxycholesterol. Also known as oxidized cholesterol, oxycholesterol is like regular cholesterol on steroids when it comes to clogging your arteries. When subjected to high heat, as in frying, grilling or broiling, cholesterol reacts with oxygen, giving rise to highly reactive oxycholesterol particles. To study how these renegade fat particles impact the health and function of arteries, scientists fed three groups of lab mice identical diets with one containing .05 percent regular cholesterol, a second .05 percent oxycholesterol and a third .1 percent oxycholesterol. The two groups consuming the oxycholesterol were hit with a litany of adverse vascular effects, including a much greater rise in cholesterol and triglyceride levels, more plaque buildup and a marked disruption in the function of the endothelial cells (cells that line arteries and control blood flow). That is a scary, quadruple insult to the "rivers of life" and some major competition for the current, artery-clogging world champion, trans fat.

Stay heart smart and keep oxycholesterol out of your body. You can do so by restricting your intake of red meats that have been fried, grilled or broiled. Keep in mind that you will never have to be concerned with this sinister substance when eating plant foods, because plants are naturally 100% cholesterol free!

A Lesson In Portion Control!

Given our overwhelming, bigger-is-better, super-sized food culture, learning how to control your portions is one of the single most powerful strategies available to you to achieve and maintain a healthy body weight. My best advice for keeping your portions on target is right in your own two hands! At meals, limit what you eat to what fits in your two hands cupped together minus any fruit and veggies (no need to limit portions of fruits or veggies). Those who engage in regular portion control have been shown to increase their chances of long-term weight loss up to 4-fold.

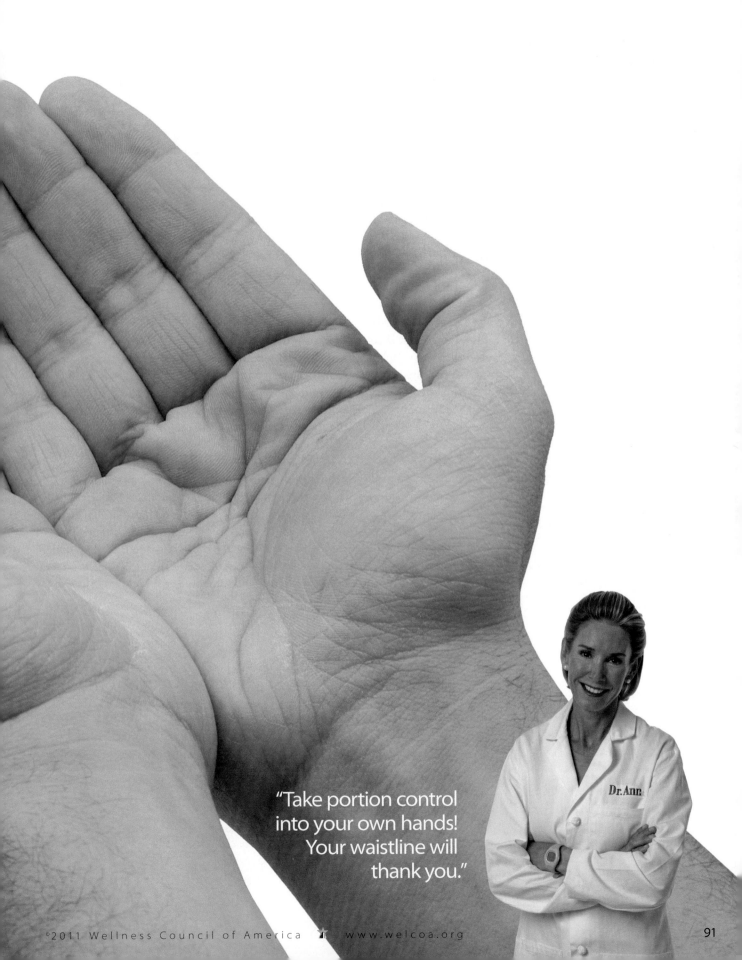

"Take portion control into your own hands! Your waistline will thank you."

Healthy Summer Grilling

Grilling is fun, easy and tasty, but may be hazardous to your health. Grilled meat, especially red meat, is a well known source of two cancer-causing agents: heterocyclic amines (HCAs) and polycyclic aromatic hydro-carbons (PAHs). HCAs develop when the muscle proteins of meats are exposed to high heat. PAHs form in the black, charred outer portions of grilled meats when their surface fats and juices come into direct contact with flame and smoke.

If you are going to grill any type of meat, you can significantly reduce your exposure to these harmful chemicals by taking the following simple steps:

- Partially pre-cook your meat in the microwave for two minutes.

- Marinate before grilling. Even a quick 30 second submersion in a marinade liquid is helpful.

- Mix some textured vegetable protein into your ground meat at a 1:9 ratio.

- Avoid well-done meats and trim away any charred portions before eating.

- Add a tablespoon or two of dried rosemary to your meat prior to grilling—it contains phytochemicals that reduce the formation of HCAs.

- Flip the meat frequently to keep the internal temperature lower.

- Stick with lean cuts and trim away as much visible fat as possible to decrease flare ups from the open flame.

- Grill meats as an occasional treat and consume moderate portions when you do.

Lastly, enjoy your grilled meat with as many brightly colored fruit and vegetable sides as possible. They provide healthful compounds that can counter-act the harmful effects of PAHs and HCAs

Full-Fat Dairy Products

Whole or full-fat dairy products are the second unhealthy protein, and I strongly recommend that you restrict these foods. Although they provide complete protein and several important nutrients, like vitamins A and D and calcium, they also provide an enormous dose of artery-clogging saturated fat and loads of calories. Whole dairy products include whole milk, regular (full-fat) cheeses, cream, ice cream, and sour cream. Always choose low-fat, reduced-fat, or skim varieties of dairy. With this simple tactic, you can reduce calories and fat and still take full advantage of dairy's complete protein, vitamins A and D, B vitamins, calcium, magnesium, potassium, and zinc. For example, if you drink an eight-ounce glass of whole milk, you will take in 150 calories and eight grams of saturated fat (the same amount as four strips of bacon!). If you choose skim, you will get even higher levels of milk's beneficial nutrients with just half a gram of bad fat and only 80 calories.

Always choose skim or one percent milk, low-fat yogurt, and reduced-fat sour cream. If you are a cheese lover, stick to the reduced-fat versions and even then, include them in moderation. Cheese is the single greatest source of saturated fat in the American diet and the leading culprit in raising blood cholesterol levels. Part-skim mozzarella sticks and cheddar and Swiss cheese made from two percent milk are widely available. Check labels carefully to be sure you are choosing these reduced-fat cheese options.

Dairy: A Double-Edged Sword

In terms of broad spectrum health, dairy products produce a mixed bag. On the positive side, regular consumption of low-fat dairy products has been associated with protection from osteoporosis, better blood pressure control, less metabolic syndrome and less colon cancer. On the negative side, studies have consistently shown that men who consume the most dairy foods develop more prostate cancer. A few studies have shown an increased risk of Parkinson's disease in men who eat the most dairy, and some studies have shown higher rates of ovarian cancer in women who consume the most dairy. A final consideration is digestibility. About 70 percent of the world's population cannot fully digest the sugar in milk called lactose. This lactose intolerance can lead to bloating, abdominal discomfort and excess gas. If you fit into this category like I do, stick to low-fat yogurt, as the good bacteria it contains have digested the lactose for you.

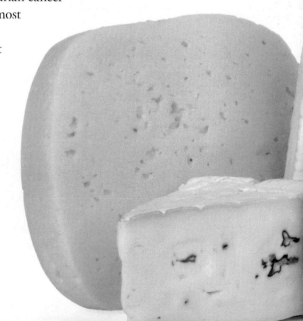

> 66 *Although they [full fat dairy products] provide complete protein and several important nutrients, like vitamins A and D and calcium, they also provide an enormous dose of artery-clogging saturated fat and loads of calories.* 99

OFFICIAL SEAL OF DISAPPROVAL
DR. ANN KULZE, MD
OFFICIAL SEAL OF DISAPPROVAL

Make The Swap

In a study involving over 29,000 post-menopausal women followed for about 15 years, those consuming the largest amount of protein from red meat and dairy had up to a 40 percent greater risk of death from heart disease versus those with the lowest intakes. Interestingly, women in this study who consumed the most vegetable-based proteins like beans and soy foods had a 30 percent lower risk of dying from heart disease than those eating the least.

Vegetable-based proteins have several distinct advantages over animal-based proteins. Replace them with animal-based proteins when you can. The richest sources of vegetable proteins include:

- **Beans and legumes:** There are over 24 varieties to choose from, including black beans, kidney beans, chickpeas, field peas, lentils and butter beans, etc.

- **Nuts:** Almonds, pecans, walnuts, cashews, hazelnuts, Brazil nuts, pine nuts and pistachios.

- **Seeds:** Pumpkin seeds, sunflower seeds, flax seeds, chia seeds, sesame seeds and hemp seeds.

- **Soy products:** Soy milk, tofu, tempeh, roasted soy nuts and edamame.

By making this swap, you can enjoy your protein along with phytochemicals, zero cholesterol, negligible to no saturated fat, a higher nutrient density and fewer calories.

Plain Yogurt: The Cream Of The Dairy Crop

As dairy foods go, low-fat plain yogurt is a superstar standout. I want you to include it in your diet regularly. Here are three big reasons why you should.

1. **Yogurt is the richest and most bio-available source of calcium.** An eight-ounce serving provides 30 to 40 percent of your daily calcium requirements. In addition to calcium, yogurt will also give you B vitamins, zinc and potassium.

2. **Yogurt contains probiotics.** Probiotics are the beneficial bacteria that reside in our colons and appear to be rapidly rising stars on the disease-fighting front. We have long known about the importance of probiotics in digestive function, but we now know that they offer additional health benefits. Probiotics have been shown to be helpful for many conditions, including inflammatory bowel disease, colic, eczema, allergies and upper respiratory infections. Mounting evidence suggests they may also aid in weight management.

3. **Yogurt is easily digested and its nutrients are better absorbed.** The good bacteria in yogurt have predigested its lactose, which means that even lactose intolerant individuals can enjoy it. These same bacteria also produce lactic acid, which aids in the absorption of calcium and B vitamins.

Ounce for ounce, low-fat plain yogurt will give you the most nutritional bang for your efforts. It has about half the calories of fruit-flavored yogurts, twice as much protein, more calcium, less fillers and no added sugar. Greek-style yogurt is now available at most grocery outlets (Oikos, FAGE) and takes health and taste to a whole new level. This special yogurt is strained to remove its liquid component, giving it a rich and creamy texture that is truly decadent. This straining process also doubles its protein and lowers its sugar (lactose) content. Here are some easy ways to bring plain yogurt into your dietary repertoire:

- Use it in place of milk in your cereal
- Make a yogurt parfait by alternating it with layers of your favorite fresh fruit
- Use it in your dips to replace mayo or sour cream
- Add it to your salad dressings for extra creaminess
- Use it in your sauces to replace butter or heavy cream
- Enjoy some all on its own as a mid-afternoon snack

If you prefer your yogurt a bit sweetened like I do, add some fresh fruit or a small portion of honey or maple syrup. And again, you should avoid fruit flavored yogurts—many contain more sugar than a standard dessert!

Learning to do your protein right is perhaps the easiest of all the *Eat Right For Life™* strategies. Here is a recap of what you need to do for success.

PLAN OF ACTION · Select the **right** proteins.

1. ALWAYS CONSUME THE HEALTHY PROTEINS

- Fish, shellfish, poultry (skinless if overweight), beans and legumes, nuts, seeds, whole soy foods, wild game, omega-3-fortified eggs and low-fat/skim dairy products are the best choices.

- Strive for three servings of fish a week. Oily fish are best (salmon, tuna, mackerel, sardines, herring and lake trout). Avoid shark, marlin, king mackerel, tile fish and swordfish due to toxins. Women of child-bearing years and children should avoid fresh tuna and canned albacore tuna.

- Consume omega-3 eggs as desired, unless you have a cholesterol problem or type 2 diabetes. These two groups should limit eggs to less than five a week.

- For optimal appetite control, be sure to include healthy proteins at each meal, especially breakfast.

2. STRIVE TO EAT MORE VEGETABLE PROTEIN

- Vegetable-based proteins guard and protect your health in ways that animal-based proteins cannot.

- Beans and legumes, nuts, seeds, nut and seed butters, and whole soy foods are all excellent sources of vegetable-based proteins. It's especially beneficial to replace the unhealthy animal proteins—beef, pork, lamb and whole dairy products—with these foods.

3. LIMIT THE UNHEALTHY PROTEINS

- Limit red meat, such as beef, pork and lamb, to two or less servings a week. Choose lean cuts when you do eat these foods. Be especially vigilant in avoiding fatty cuts and processed red meats like bacon, sausage and bologna.

- Limit or eliminate whole dairy products (whole milk, full-fat cheeses, ice cream, cream and sour cream). Opt for the low-fat versions instead.

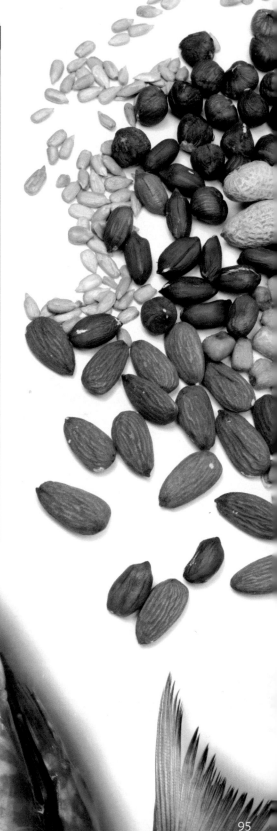

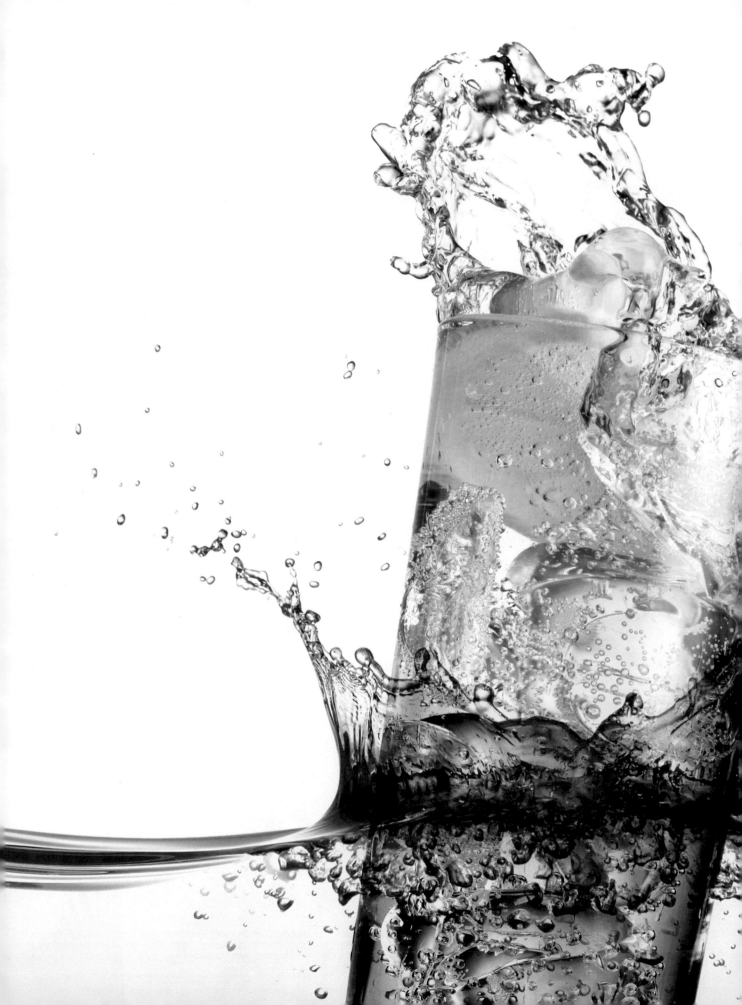

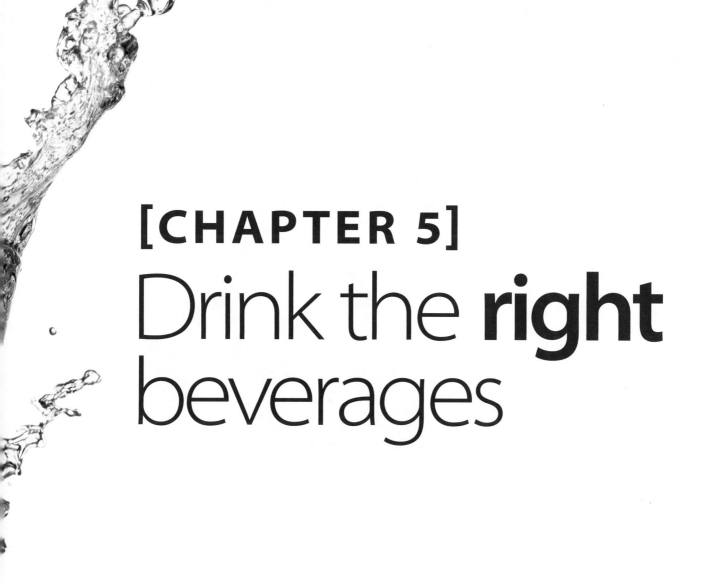

[CHAPTER 5]
Drink the **right** beverages

[CHAPTER 5]

Drink the **right** beverages

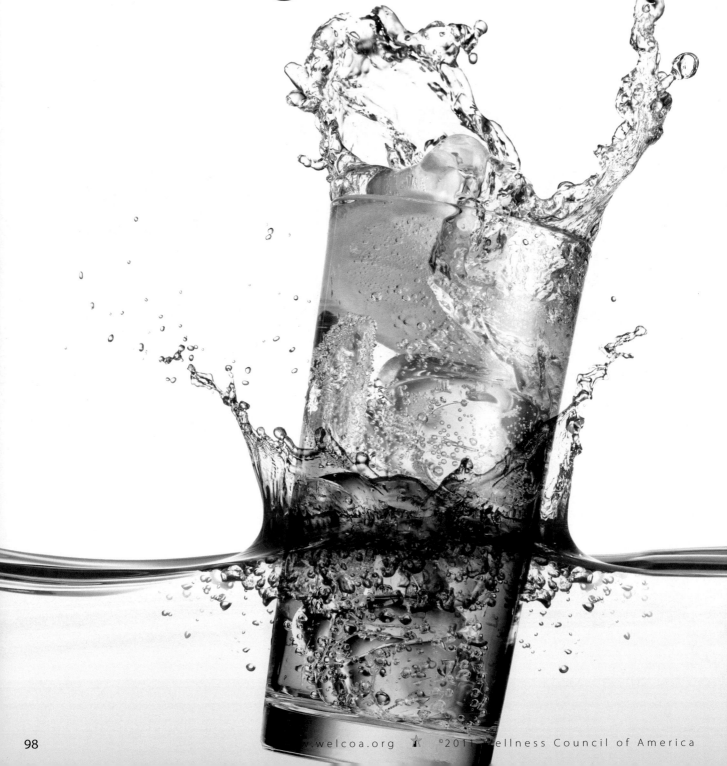

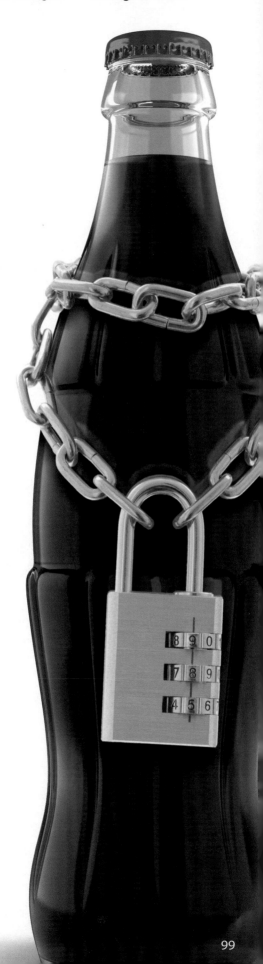

Although I wrote this book to educate and guide you in the healthiest way to eat, I would be completely remiss if I didn't offer some guidance on beverages. At this time, beverages constitute a whopping 22 percent of the total daily calories consumed in America. This glaring statistic underscores just how crucial it is to do your beverages right.

As you will learn in a moment, what you choose to drink can have a profound impact on your health and your body weight. To maximize your liquid intake, I'm going to walk you through the beverages you need to dump and the beverages you need to gulp. We'll cover the drinks you need to dump first.

THE DRINKS YOU NEED TO DUMP

All Sugary Drinks

Of all the things you can do to improve your wellness and meet your weight goals, dumping your liquid calories likely offers the single greatest return for your efforts. Over the past several years, liquid calories, especially sugary beverages, have emerged as the most fattening or weight-boosting of all types of calories. Whether you are partial to soda, sports drinks or fruit drinks, each time you quench your thirst with one of these popular beverages, you consume calories derived entirely from sugar. These liquid sugars have a very high glycemic response because they can bypass the digestive process altogether and zip straight into your bloodstream as a flash flood of glucose and fructose. The fallout from these notorious "twin peaks" is metabolic stress that can have far-reaching consequences throughout the body.

How Sugary Drinks Make Us Fat

Tragically, sugary beverages are now the number one source of calories in the toxic U.S. diet. Scientific studies consistently link the intake of sweet beverages to weight gain, obesity, type 2 diabetes and metabolic syndrome. In fact, sugary beverages tend to be particularly obesigenic because they lack physical bulk and do not suppress the appetite to the same degree as solid-food calories. They simply do not fill the stomach and elicit the cascade of hunger-suppressing signals that solid foods do.

Every sip of these sweet beverages immediately raises blood glucose and blood fructose levels. This "double-whammy" triggers hunger and promotes fat storage. Lastly, drinking rather than chewing provides less opportunity for satisfying the cravings of your mouth and makes it considerably easier to take in excess calories quickly and effortlessly.

Indeed, sugary beverages provide a perfect storm of easy calories that do nothing to satisfy your hunger. Consider this: if you drink one 16-ounce soda daily (that's 200 calories) over and above the calories you expend, you will gain 20 pounds in one year. Stated another way, if you stop drinking that 16-ounce bottle of soda and otherwise maintain your current level of calorie intake, you can lose up to 20 pounds in one year.

The unique propensity of sugary beverages to promote weight gain has been well-documented in the research. In a report from the Harvard Nurses' Health Study, investigators followed the drinking habits of over 51,000 women from 1991 to 1995. Over the four-year period, study subjects who increased their intake of sugary beverages to one or more a day increased their calories by 358 per day. This same group gained over 10 pounds over the four-year study interval.

When we drink sugary beverages, we simply do not compensate for these liquid calories by eating less food. Scientists from Penn State fed 33 adult subjects lunch with a non-caloric beverage like water or a caloric beverage like soda. The researchers determined that people consumed just as much food when they drank soda and ultimately consumed 128 to 151 more calories at the lunch test meal versus the exact same test meal served with water. They also found that the larger the beverage serving size, the more the study subjects drank. So, take note: those unlimited soda refills frequently offered in restaurants are a surefire recipe for weight gain.

Lastly, a recent landmark clinical trial determined how changes in liquid calories affect body weight, and I hope the results will spur you to dump sugary beverages once and for all. Known as the "PREMIER Trial," this study confirmed that reducing liquid calories by as little as 100 calories a day (half a bottle of soda) led to significant weight loss by the end of the 18-month study period. This study also determined that reducing liquid calories has a larger impact on weight reduction than reducing the equivalent amount of solid food calories. Moreover, previous scientific observations have found that reducing liquid calories does not seem to make us hungrier (as is the case with cutting back on solid food calories). These collective findings ultimately tell me that dumping your liquid calories is the easiest and the most powerful means to weight loss.

www.welcoa.org ★ ©2011 Wellness Council of America

Soda: Just Say No

I stand firmly on record as a wellness expert who strongly discourages the consumption of all sugar-fortified beverages, especially soda. In fact, of all the radical and adverse changes in the modern American diet, our record consumption of liquid sugars is arguably the most profound. Aside from smoking, consuming sugary beverages tops my list of unhealthy habits. As a form of unhealthy calories, soda is simply in a league of its own. Soda has ZERO nutritional value and has repeatedly and consistently been associated with great harm. Here are some key research findings:

- Women who increased soda consumption to one a day increased their risk of type 2 diabetes 83 percent compared to those consuming one or less monthly.

- For kids, each additional daily serving of soda increased the risk of obesity by 60 percent.

- A single daily serving of soda caused significant tooth enamel erosion. Four cups a day increased the risk by 252 percent.

- Adults who consumed two or more sodas per week were 87 percent more likely to develop pancreatic cancer (one of the most lethal cancers) than those who didn't drink soda.

- Those who drank the most soda consumed less milk, essential nutrients, fruit and fiber. They did, however, consume more carbohydrate calories.

- Those drinking two or more colas a day more than doubled their risk of chronic kidney disease.

- Those drinking one or more soft drinks a day were 44 percent more likely to develop metabolic syndrome than those who drank less than one a day.

- Women who consumed two or more sweetened beverages daily were 35 percent more likely to have a heart attack versus those who drank one or less a month.

Need I say more—just say no to soda!

(Continued on page 104)

Soda: Bad To The Bone

All carbonated beverages, including diet brands, are acidic in nature. The acids from carbonated beverages enter your bloodstream and are buffered by calcium. However, if the calcium levels in the bloodstream are inadequate, your bones will supply it. Studies have shown that even modest levels of cola consumption are associated with lower bone mineral density scores. And our teeth fare even worse than our bones. The acids in soda damage tooth enamel. As little as a single cup serving of soda a day has been shown to cause significant, irreversible tooth enamel erosion.

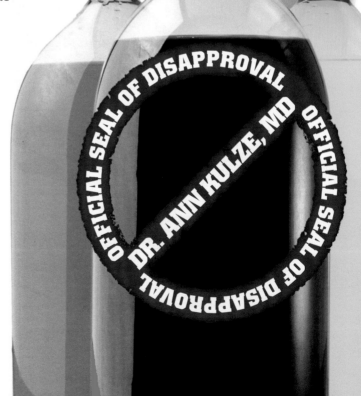

FAST FACT:

Most sugary beverages contain the equivalent of 11–12 teaspoons of sugar per bottle.

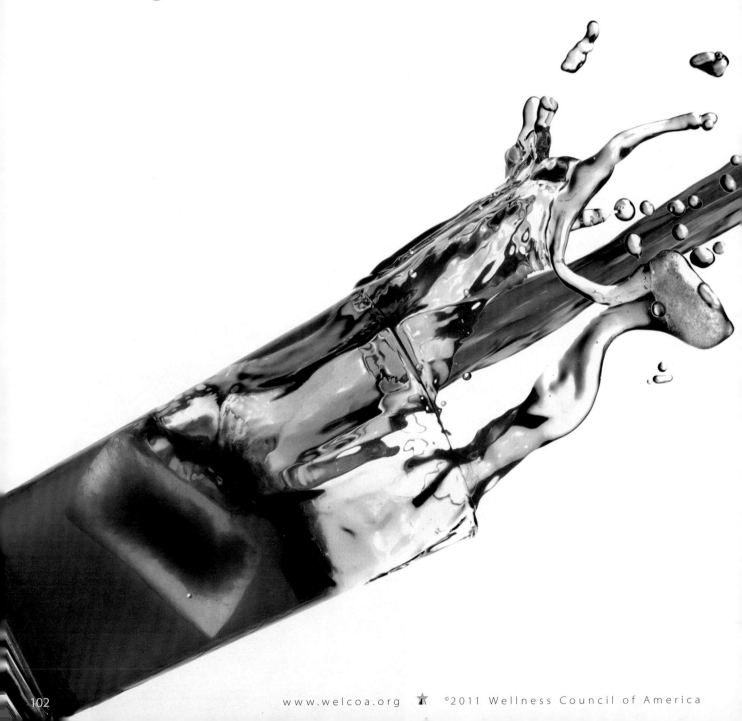

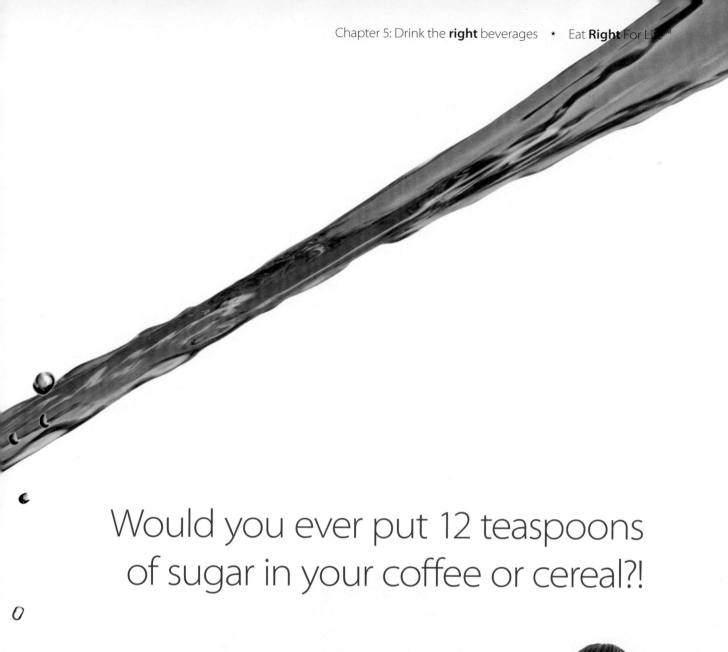

Would you ever put 12 teaspoons of sugar in your coffee or cereal?!

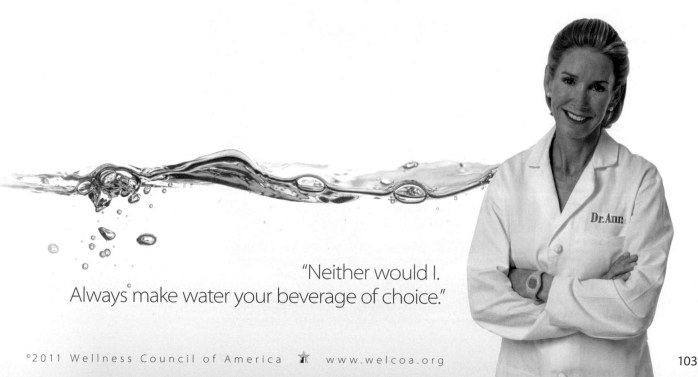

"Neither would I.
Always make water your beverage of choice."

> *If insulin is released with no real glucose coming in, blood sugar levels will drop, which can incite hunger.*

What About Diet Drinks?

Alas, I must tell you that diet sodas are an unacceptable alternative. I strongly discourage both regular and diet soda. I imagine that you may be wondering how this seemingly benign, zero calorie beverage could do any harm. Although I do think diet soda is clearly the lesser of two evils, emerging data has suggested that this trendy beverage may indeed come with some health risks.

The famed Framington Heart Study found that study participants who consumed one or more diet sodas a day experienced a 50 to 60 percent greater risk of developing metabolic syndrome. Metabolic syndrome is an epidemic condition in which a person has at least three cardiovascular risk factors occurring simultaneously. As you would expect, it dramatically boosts the risk of heart disease. In fact, about 60 percent of all heart attacks can be directly attributed to it. A second report found that cola lovers—including those who drank diet versions—could be harming their kidneys. In this evaluation, subjects who consumed two or more servings of diet cola daily were almost two and a half times more likely to develop kidney disease. The study's authors speculate that a common preservative (phosphoric acid) is the likely culprit. High levels of phosphoric acid are a recognized irritant for the kidneys.

Believe it or not, these so-called "diet" drinks may actually result in weight gain, despite their zero calorie make-up. Animal studies have found that artificial sweeteners can interfere with the body's natural ability to match caloric intake to energy expenditure. Additionally, the mere taste of something sweet in our mouths may trigger a blood insulin response. If insulin is released with no real glucose coming in, blood sugar levels will drop, which can incite hunger.

Anecdotally, I've had several people in my private wellness coaching practice lose weight by simply giving up their daily diet sodas. If you are hooked on diet sodas, work on weaning yourself from them; they are simply not healthy beverages. If you miss the caffeine kick, substitute soda with some freshly brewed unsweetened tea.

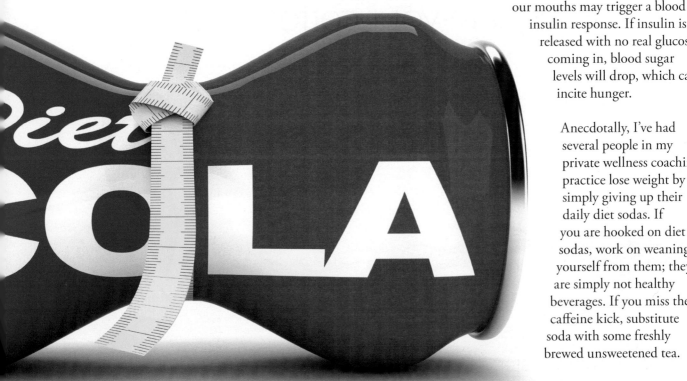

Keeping It Real

With the exception of those with diabetes, I do not recommend the use of artificial sweeteners. Although science supports their long-term safety, I am concerned that they may lead to weight gain. There are several biologically plausible mechanisms whereby this could take place. A provocative laboratory study recently provided some hard evidence to support my fears. Purdue University researchers fed one group of rats artificially sweetened yogurt and a second group sugar-sweetened yogurt. Rats getting the artificially sweetened yogurt ate more food and gained more weight than rats eating sugar-sweetened yogurt. As demonstrated in previous laboratory studies, artificial sweeteners can interfere with the body's natural ability to use sensory cues to gauge calorie consumption. Artificial sweeteners are exquisitely sweet substances—anywhere from 40 to 800 times sweeter than table sugar—yet they have no calories. When included regularly in the diet, the body may not expect much in terms of calories from sweets, and respond by ultimately eating more! At a minimum, I can assure you that artificial sweeteners exploit the human palate's highly developed taste for sweets. If you include them regularly, the bar for what tastes sweet is going to be set stratospherically high. In this situation, I have concerns that you will never be able to appreciate and be satisfied with the delicious and healthy sweetness of nature's dessert, namely fruit.

Assuming you are not diabetic, when you feel the need to sweeten a food or beverage (which shouldn't be very often or in large quantities), just use a little bit of the real thing. I put a teaspoon of real sugar or honey in my morning coffee and I'm still lean and healthy. In the context of a healthy diet and adequate levels of physical activity, a small amount of sugar is not harmful.

> *...artificial sweeteners exploit the human palate's highly developed taste for sweets.*

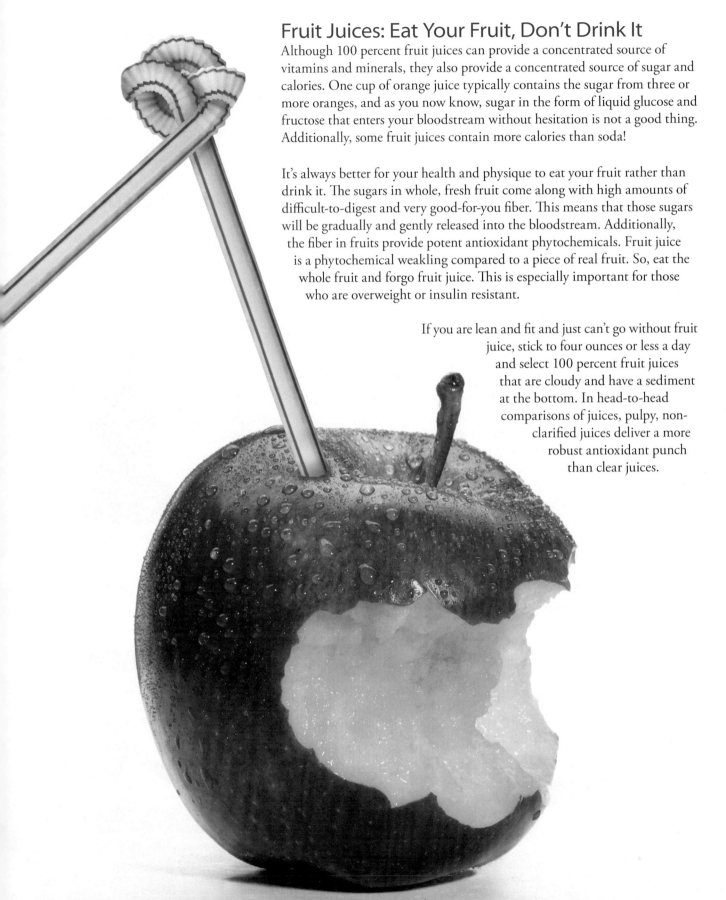

Fruit Juices: Eat Your Fruit, Don't Drink It

Although 100 percent fruit juices can provide a concentrated source of vitamins and minerals, they also provide a concentrated source of sugar and calories. One cup of orange juice typically contains the sugar from three or more oranges, and as you now know, sugar in the form of liquid glucose and fructose that enters your bloodstream without hesitation is not a good thing. Additionally, some fruit juices contain more calories than soda!

It's always better for your health and physique to eat your fruit rather than drink it. The sugars in whole, fresh fruit come along with high amounts of difficult-to-digest and very good-for-you fiber. This means that those sugars will be gradually and gently released into the bloodstream. Additionally, the fiber in fruits provide potent antioxidant phytochemicals. Fruit juice is a phytochemical weakling compared to a piece of real fruit. So, eat the whole fruit and forgo fruit juice. This is especially important for those who are overweight or insulin resistant.

If you are lean and fit and just can't go without fruit juice, stick to four ounces or less a day and select 100 percent fruit juices that are cloudy and have a sediment at the bottom. In head-to-head comparisons of juices, pulpy, non-clarified juices deliver a more robust antioxidant punch than clear juices.

THE DRINKS YOU NEED TO GULP
Water: The Perfect Beverage

There is one, and only one, beverage that is perfectly suited to our biological needs: pure, clean, natural water. Water is the body's most vital essential nutrient. Illness and death will ensue from lack of water much more quickly than any other essential nutrient. Water best suits the liquid requirements of the human body—it has zero calories and is free of unhealthy additives.

On average, water makes up 65 percent of the body and it performs a variety of vital functions. It helps regulate body temperature, cushions internal organs, lubricates joints, keeps our mucous membranes moist, and is the medium in which virtually every chemical and metabolic reaction in the body occurs. The amount of water you need to drink is based on how many calories you burn daily. The U.S. Recommended Daily Allowance for water is one milliliter per calorie burned. If you expend 2,000 calories a day, you require 2,000 milliliters, or two liters of water a day. This figure must be increased for physical activity, hot or humid environments, high altitudes, illness, pregnancy and nursing. The average woman needs 2.7 liters daily and the average man requires 3.7 liters.

Always make water your beverage of choice. Drink water with your meals and always try to keep some within arm's reach to take the edge off your thirst. For those who currently drink sugary beverages and need to lose weight, I want to remind you that substituting water is the most powerful and effective change you can make to improve your chances of weight loss success. I have seen countless patients successfully lose weight just by substituting water for sodas and other sugar-fortified beverages. So ditch the soda and make the switch!

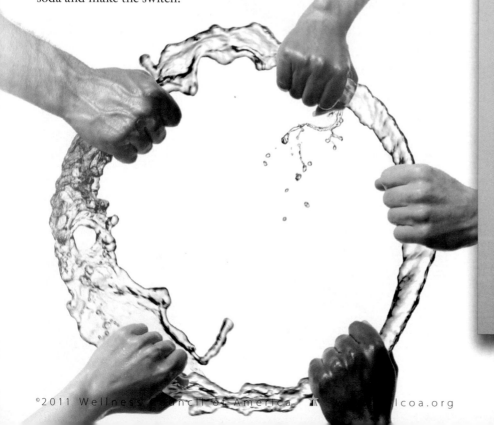

Is Bottled Water Better?

It is an urban myth that bottled water is healthier than tap water. Municipal water supplies are more rigorously tested and monitored than bottled waters, and tap water costs a fraction of a cent (which is at least 200 times cheaper than bottled water). Additionally, many bottled waters come straight from the tap anyway. If you have any concerns about the safety or quality of your tap water, consider purchasing a home water purification system.

Moreover, please don't waste your money on the dizzying array of "fortified" waters now commonly available on grocery store shelves. There is no evidence that taking in vitamins, minerals or other "healthy" additives in this manner has any health benefits. To the contrary, given the growing number of fortified foods and popular use of supplements, I have concerns that some people may be consuming too much of them. With vitamins and minerals, more is not necessarily better, and can even be dangerous. Lastly, many of these designer waters are loaded with sugar, and you know by now that sugary beverages are unhealthy and should be avoided. Don't be duped and do not waste your money on these products.

(Continued on page 110)

FAST FACT:

Americans now drink an enormous amount of liquid sugar calories that averages to 300 calories a day!

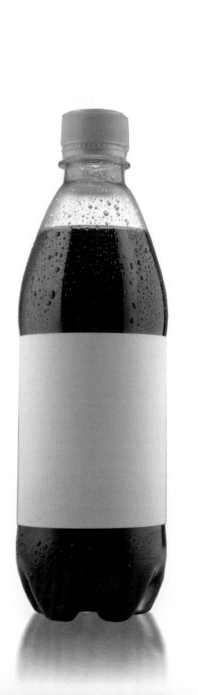
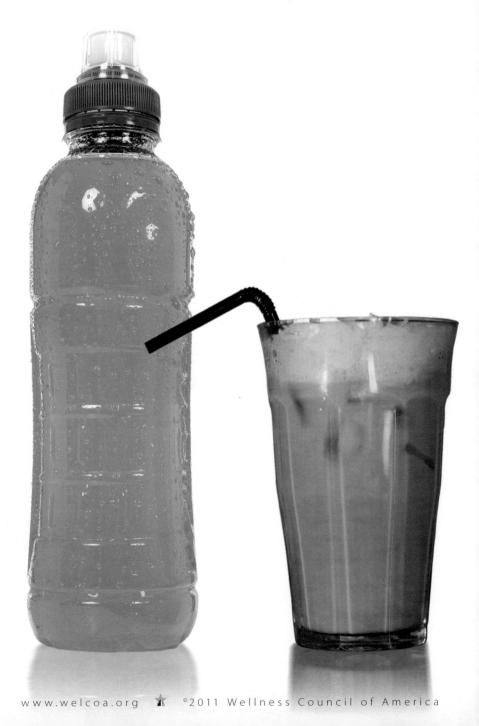

If Americans stopped drinking sugary beverages, it would likely halt the obesity epidemic dead in its tracks.

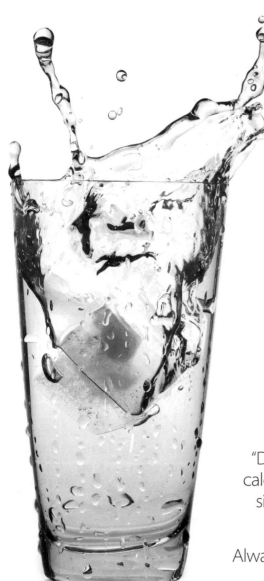

"Dumping your liquid calories likely offers the single greatest return on your health.

Always make water your beverage of choice."

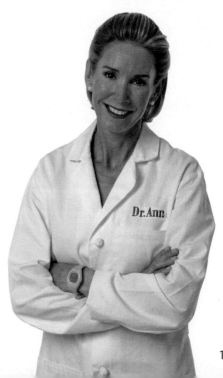

"All forms of freshly brewed tea are great for you—green, black, white and oolong."

Vegetable Juice: An Exception To The Juice Rule

While studies consistently show that drinking calories provides less appetite suppression than eating them, vegetable juice may be the exception. Including vegetable juice in your diet is a good idea for a variety of reasons. It's brimming with vitamins A and C and potassium as well as numerous other health-boosting nutrients and antioxidants. A single, four-ounce glass of vegetable juice counts as a full serving of vegetables. Relative to most other beverages, 100 percent vegetable juice is low in calories and will not spike your blood glucose and fructose levels. In fact, drinking a glass of vegetable juice prior to a meal appears to help us eat less. Researchers at Baylor College of Medicine had 81 study participants drink zero, one, or two eight-ounce cups of low sodium vegetable juice daily for 12 weeks. Those who drank the vegetable juice lost an average of four pounds during the 12 weeks, while those who didn't lost just one pound. Scientists speculate that the fiber or perhaps the concentrated supply of nutrients found in vegetable juice may take the edge off hunger.

Tea: Brewing With Benefits

Freshly brewed tea can decrease your cardiovascular risk, boost your immunity, slow your cognitive decline, kick up your metabolism, help mitigate stress and likely reduce your cancer risk—all for zero calories! Based on the science and my own personal experience, I am wildly enthusiastic about regularly drinking freshly brewed, unsweetened tea. This superstar elixir of good health is exploding with potent antioxidants called catechins. These special chemicals protect our bodies from the ravages of free radicals even more effectively than the antioxidants in fruits and veggies. If you are not currently taking advantage of freshly brewed tea, you should start today. I sip on freshly brewed, unsweetened tea throughout my work day and find it the easiest, quickest and most relaxing way to continuously infuse my body and brain with those life-preserving antioxidants.

All forms of freshly brewed tea are great for you—green, black, white and oolong. They are all derived from the same leaf, the camellia sinensis leaf (home to those remarkable antioxidant catechins). Drink the varieties you enjoy—cold or hot, bagged or loose-leaf—just brew it yourself to fully exploit its goodness. The processing required for powdered, bottled or decaffeinated teas destroys many of its antioxidants. Further, the bottled and powdered versions usually have added sugars or artificial sweeteners, which is another drawback.

For best results, steep your tea of choice for at least three minutes and squeeze the bag at the end of steeping to extract as many remaining catechins as possible. Avoid added milk or cream, as studies have shown they bind tea's beneficial compounds, rendering them unavailable to work their antioxidant magic for the body. Do add a twist of lemon or lime though. A recent report found that the vitamin C in citrus enhances the absorption of catechins up to three-fold!

Alcohol: Benefits In Moderation

Given the popularity of this particular beverage, I think it's important to provide you with the latest scientific facts on alcohol and health. Including alcohol in moderation, defined as one drink or less a day for women and two drinks or less a day for men, lowers the risk of heart disease and ischemic strokes by about 30 percent. Over 100 studies have supported these findings. A growing number of studies have shown that a little bit of alcohol on a daily basis can improve insulin sensitivity, which may lower the risk of type 2 diabetes and improve weight control. Including alcohol in moderation has also been linked to protection from dementia and greater overall longevity. However, there is a very fine line when it comes to alcohol use and reaping potential health benefits. As soon as you cross over from moderate to higher levels, even slightly higher levels, disease risk quickly mounts. We have conclusive evidence that drinking excess alcohol increases the risk of many cancers, damages the brain, liver and heart, increases blood pressure, incites bleeding strokes and leads to addiction and accidents.

As a female with a family history of breast cancer, I want to be certain that women know that alcohol is the single most powerful nutritional risk factor for breast cancer. Even going from one drink a day to two has been shown in several studies to boost breast cancer risk by 25 to 30 percent. Binge drinking is especially risky for breast health. If you are concerned about breast cancer, alcohol should be avoided.

The decision to drink in moderation or not to drink should be individualized and should consider your personal and family medical history. If you enjoy alcohol and do not have a medical condition in which alcohol has been prohibited, including a drink a day can be harmonious with healthy living.

Red wine has special features that deserve mention. Because it is fermented with the grapes and their skins, red wine is exceptionally high in powerful antioxidants called polyphenols. A growing number of studies suggest that red wine may have benefits over and above other forms of alcohol—likely because of its superior antioxidant status. Red wines can vary dramatically in their levels of beneficial antioxidants. According to an analysis published in *Nature*, red wines from Sardinia and South Western France have up to five to ten times more polyphenols than wines produced elsewhere. A small glass of red wine with dinner would be the healthiest way to include alcohol.

Hold The Red Wine—That Is… In Your Mouth

Resveratrol, a super-strong antioxidant in red wine, has become somewhat of a wonder compound in the laboratory. Studies have linked it with a host of remarkable benefits from cancer prevention to slowing the aging process. Unfortunately, resveratrol is very poorly absorbed once it enters the gastrointestinal tract. New research, however, has shown that it can be readily absorbed through the mucous membranes lining our mouths. One study reported blood levels of resveratrol up to 100 times greater if the red wine was slowly sipped and allowed to linger in the mouth versus being gulped down. So for best results, sip and savor!

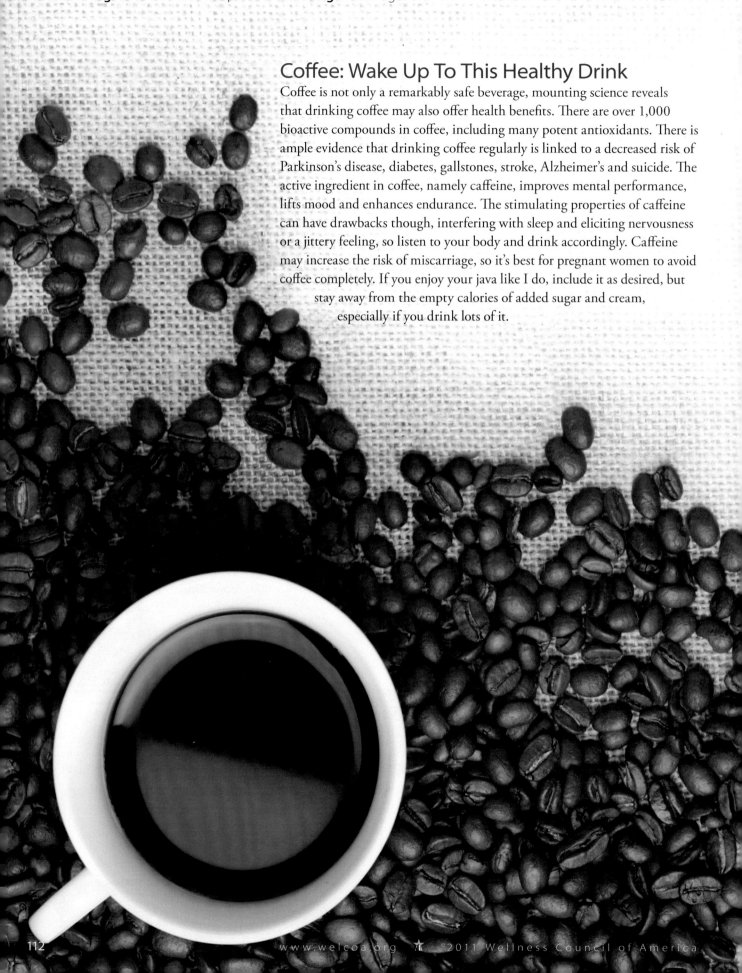

Coffee: Wake Up To This Healthy Drink

Coffee is not only a remarkably safe beverage, mounting science reveals that drinking coffee may also offer health benefits. There are over 1,000 bioactive compounds in coffee, including many potent antioxidants. There is ample evidence that drinking coffee regularly is linked to a decreased risk of Parkinson's disease, diabetes, gallstones, stroke, Alzheimer's and suicide. The active ingredient in coffee, namely caffeine, improves mental performance, lifts mood and enhances endurance. The stimulating properties of caffeine can have drawbacks though, interfering with sleep and eliciting nervousness or a jittery feeling, so listen to your body and drink accordingly. Caffeine may increase the risk of miscarriage, so it's best for pregnant women to avoid coffee completely. If you enjoy your java like I do, include it as desired, but stay away from the empty calories of added sugar and cream, especially if you drink lots of it.

Use the following *Drink The Right Beverages Plan Of Action* to guide you in choosing the best beverages for your health and wellness.

PLAN OF ACTION Drink the **right** beverages.

1. **DRINK PURE, CLEAN WATER AS YOUR BEVERAGE OF CHOICE.**

2. **AVOID ALL SUGARY BEVERAGES: SODA (INCLUDING DIET), FRUIT DRINKS, CHOCOLATE MILK, SUGAR-SWEETENED TEA, SPORTS DRINKS*, DESSERT COFFEE BEVERAGES AND ANY OTHER SUGAR-FORTIFIED BEVERAGES. SUGARY BEVERAGES HAVE BEEN SHOWN TO PROMOTE WEIGHT GAIN (WHICH PROMOTES MOST DISEASES), OBESITY, TYPE 2 DIABETES, METABOLIC SYNDROME AND TOOTH DECAY.**

3. **IN ADDITION TO WATER, PERMISSIBLE BEVERAGES INCLUDE:**

- 100 percent vegetable or tomato juice. Vegetable/tomato juice prior to a meal may be especially helpful for those who need to lose weight. Low sodium varieties are best.

- If you are lean and active, 100 percent fruit juice can be included in moderation. Limit to four ounces a day. Strictly avoid if overweight, diabetic or insulin resistant.

- Organic, plain soy milk

- One percent or skim organic milk

- Unsweetened, freshly brewed tea (green, black, white or oolong). Strive for two or more cups daily. Add a twist of citrus to kick up the flavor and to enhance absorption of its antioxidants. Herbal teas are fine too.

- Coffee as tolerated. Unsweetened, black or with skim milk is best. (Avoid if pregnant)

- For those who enjoy alcohol and have no personal medical history to preclude its safe use, alcohol can be included in moderation (if in doubt, discuss with your healthcare provider). One drink or less a day for women and two drinks or less a day for men. One drink equals 12 ounces of beer, one-and-a-half ounces of hard liquor, or five ounces of wine. Red wine is best. Make any beer low carb.

- (*Sports beverages are acceptable in the context of strenuous physical activity lasting more than one hour.)

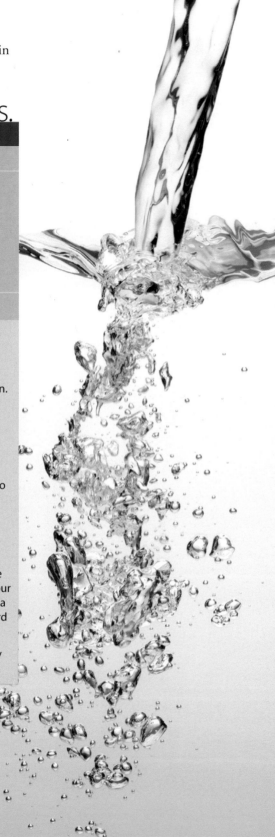

[IN SUMMARY]
Your "life plan"

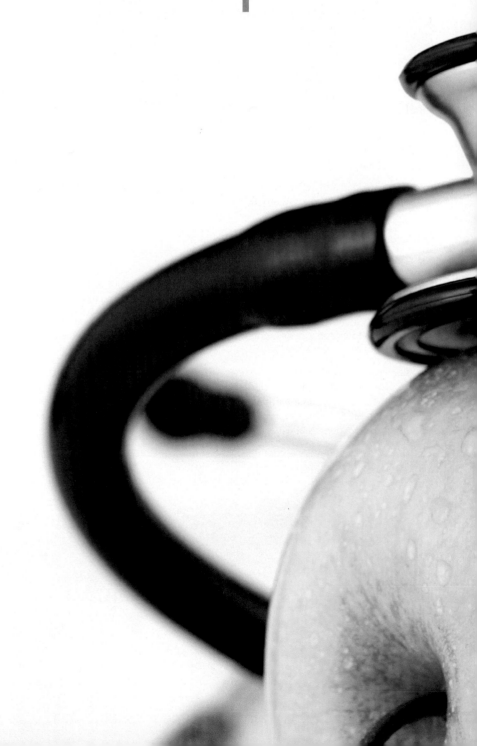

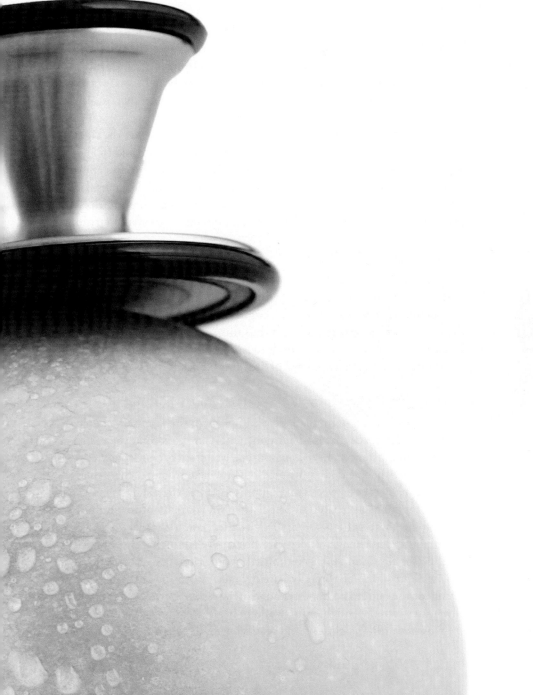

done **right**

Your "life plan" done **right**

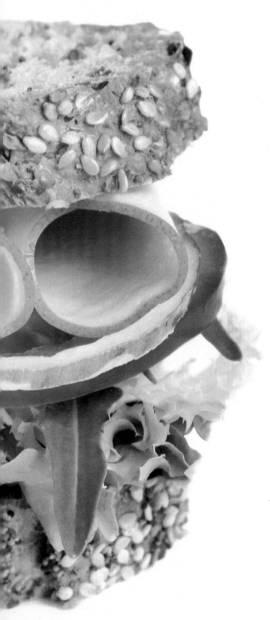

Thank you so much for allowing me to share the pleasures of healthy eating with you. I consider it an honor to guide you down the road to a healthier life and can hope for nothing less than your complete and total success. Over the years, I have been blessed with the opportunity to witness scores of people totally transform their health and quality of life simply by changing the foods they eat, and I know you can do it too. I continue to remain in awe of the astounding power the right foods have in their abilities to provide both sensory pleasure and to keep the human body in excellent working order. Before leaving you to embark on this amazing journey into a world of healthy foods and delicious flavors, I want to share some parting words of wisdom that you will find helpful as you aspire to fully experience the glorious goodness of optimal nourishment.

This Is A "Life Plan"

Keep in mind that what I have provided you with is a "life plan" and not a "diet." Each and every one of the directives we covered are things that you should strive to do forever. The original meaning of the Latin root for the word "diet" is "way of life," and thus this "diet" should be taken as a blueprint for optimal nutrition built to last a lifetime. Remember, the right foods can be your greatest source of life, joy and health.

Move To The Beat Of Your Own Drum

Because this is a long-term plan, please implement the necessary changes in your diet at a pace that is in harmony with your life's context and personal circumstances. In my one-on-one wellness coaching practice, I find that most people do best by making anywhere from 1-3 changes at a time. It usually takes 3 weeks to 6 months for a healthy dietary change to become ingrained as a habit, so be persistent in your commitment until it has become a way of life for you. Once you feel confident that you have a change or several changes under your belt, move triumphantly on to the next. Personally, I am 200% committed to nutritional excellence and don't just "walk my talk," but literally "run my talk." I continue to tweak my own eating for the better and honestly hope my wellness journey never ends. My adventures into the enlightening world of healthy eating have been amongst the most rewarding, delicious and gratifying of all of my life's experiences.

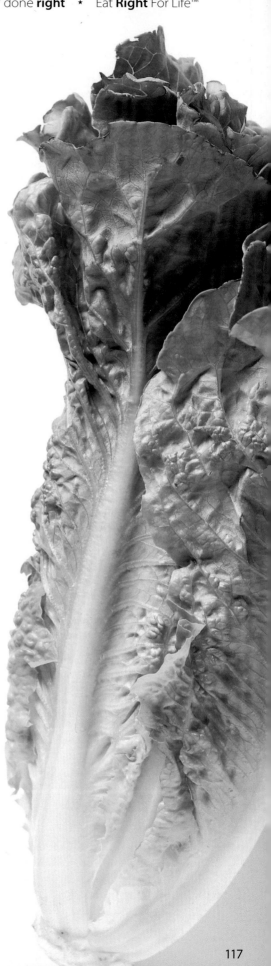

You Don't Have To Be Perfect

One of the greatest gifts of eating right is that when you occasionally fall off the wagon, you need not worry. As long as you are true to healthy eating most of the time, your body can readily compensate for intermittent indiscretions. Developing an unrestrained, positive relationship with food is a welcome natural by-product of eating healthfully.

Look Forward To Taste Bud Transformation

As you gradually change out the wrong foods for the right foods, your taste buds will change too. Healthy foods will taste better and better, and unhealthy foods will not taste as good as they used too. This may sound too good to be true, but I hear it repeatedly—statements like, "Sweets are sickeningly sweet now" or "Fast food makes me feel so bad that it tastes bad too." Trust me, you will begin to crave the taste of the good stuff like dark, leafy greens just like I do. It is a beautiful thing!

Even Baby Steps Count Big

Even the smallest improvements you can make in accordance with this dietary way of life can pay significant dividends. Celebrate each and every success and let it fuel your confidence that you can dramatically change your health and quality of life for the better simply by putting the right foods in your mouth.

Share Your New Found Nutritional Wisdom With Others

Perhaps the very best way for you to "learn" and fully internalize how to Eat Right For Life™ is to teach someone else. I encourage you to go to my website **www.DrAnnwellness.com** and download the free "cliff notes" version of this book and literally memorize the nuts and bolts of this plan so you can teach those that you love. Everything you need to know fits on a single sheet front and back! If you want an even shorter study guide, download my free Live Life! Scorecard which can be found at **www.DrAnnWellness.com**.

Please Visit Me

My website is now my busiest office and I have a 24/7 open door policy! I have created a full library of free wellness resources to help you live your healthiest life and encourage you to take full advantage of them. They include: video tips of the most frequently asked questions, detailed weekly dinner menus based on what I feed my own family, my monthly e-newsletter, free articles, my blog, plus more. If you want to get really personal with me, join me on Twitter at **DrAnnWellness**.

Lastly, never forget that YOU are the only person that can make YOU healthy, and nothing is more fundamental to a happy, productive and fulfilling life than having and owning your own health. I wish you the best of health and will always be cheering you on!

Citations

Do your fats right

Journal of the American Medical Association 6:295, 2006
New England Journal of Medicine 21:337, 1997
Circulation 14:115, 2007
66th Scientific Session of American Diabetes Association, June 2006
Annual Meeting for the Society for Neuro Science, San Diego, October 2004
Journal of the American College of Cardiology 4:48, 2006
The American Journal of Clinical Nutrition 3:90, 2009
Cell Metabolism 4:8, 2008
Gastroenterology 25:133, 2007
Lyon Heart Study 1988
The Lancet 343:8911, 1994
Journal of the American Medical Association 20:288, 2002
The Archives of Ophthalmology 12:121, 2003
American Journal of Clinical Nutrition 3:88, 2008
Circulation 106:2747, 2002
Journal of Psychiatry 8:164, 2007
American Journal of Clinical Nutrition 6:85, 2007
Archives of Neurology 11:63, 2006
American Journal of Clinical Nutrition 4:85, 2007
The Journal of Clinical Investigation 10:115, 2005
World Review Nutr Diet 66, 1991
American Journal of Clinical Nutrition 5:85, 2007
American Journal of Clinical Nutrition 5:69, 1999
Journal of the American College of Cardiology 7:54, 2009

Do your carbs right

Pediatrics 3:103, 1999
American Journal of Epidemiology 4:161 2005
Morbidity and Mortality Weekly Report 53, 2004
The American Journal of Clinical Nutrition 6:71, 2000
The American Journal of Clinical Nutrition 3:87, 2008
Journal of the American Medical Association 6:227, 1997
Diabetes Care11:27, 2004
The American Journal of Clinical Nutrition 3:87, 2008,
Journal of the National Cancer Institute 3:96, 2004
New England Journal of Medicine 17:348, 2003
Journal of Agricultural and Food Chemistry 27:51, 2003
Archives of Internal Medicine 21:161, 2001
American Journal of Clinical Nutrition 1:87, 2008
238th National Meeting of the American Chemical Society, August, 2009
Nutrition, Metabolism and Cardiovascular Diseases 4:18, 2007
American Journal of Clinical Nutrition 1:83, 2007
Nutrition and Cancer 2:30, 1998
American Journal of Clinical Nutrition 1:87, 2008
American Journal of Clinical Nutrition 3:87, 2008

Eat your fruits and veggies

Journal of the National Cancer Institute 23:87, 1995
Proceedings of the National Academy of Sciences Online Sept. 8th, 2009
Journal of the National Cancer Institute 21:96, 2004
American Journal of Clinical Nutrition 3:76, 2002
Food, Nutrition, Physical Activity, and the Prevention of Cancer, AICR, 2007
PLoS ONE 3:7, 2008
Neurology 8:67, 2006
Ophthalmology 5:116, 2009
Archives of Ophthalmology 6:122, 2004
American Journal of Clinical Nutrition 6:85, 2007
North American Association for the Study of Obesity Meeting, Las Vegas, November 2004

Select the right proteins

Journal of the American College of Cardiology 6:52, 2008
JAMA 24:288, 2002
Neurology 6:71, 2008
American Journal of Clinical Nutrition 2:90, 2009
Archives of Internal Medicine 10:167, 2007
PLos Medicine 4:12, 2007
54th Annual Meeting of the American College of Sports Medicine, New Orleans, LA., June 2007
Archives of Internal Medicine 6:169, 2009
Cancer Epidemiology Biomarkers and Prevention 5:10, 2001
Diabetes Care, September 9:27, 2004
New England Journal of Medicine 1:350, 2004
American Chemical Society Meeting, Washington, DC, Aug 09
American Journal of Epidemiology 3:161, 2005
American Journal of Clinical Nutrition 1:82 2005
American Journal of Epidemiology 5:143, 1996
Annals of Internal Medicine 6:138, 2003

Drink the right beverages

JAMA 8:292 2004
American Journal of Clinical Nutrition 5:89, 2009
Circulation 5:116, 2007
Epidemiology 4:18 2007
JAMA 8:292, 2004
The Lancet 9255:357, 2001
British Dental Journal 5:196, 2004
Epidemiology, Biomarkers and Prevention 2:19, 2010
American Journal of Public Health 4:97, 2007
Circulation 5:16, 2007
American Journal of Clinical Nutrition 4: 89, 2009
Experimental Biology Meeting, New Orleans, La., April 2009
Nature 7119:444, 2006

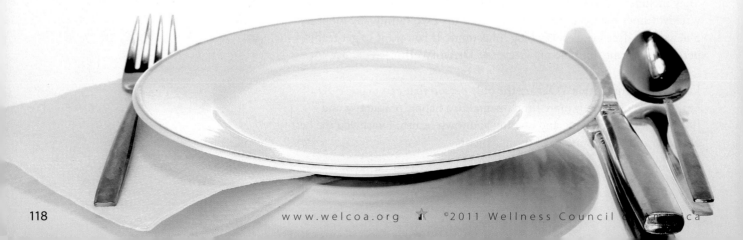